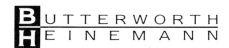
BUTTERWORTH
HEINEMANN

OXFORD   AUCKLAND   BOSTON   JOHANNESBURG   MELBOURNE   NEW DELHI

Butterworth-Heinemann
Linacre House, Jordan Hill, Oxford OX2 8DP
225 Wildwood Avenue, Woburn, MA 01801-2041
A division of Reed Educational and Professional Publishing Ltd

A member of the Reed Elsevier plc group

First published 2002

British Library Cataloguing in Publication Data
A catalogue record for this book is available from the British Library

Library of Congress Cataloguing in Publication Data
A catalogue record for this book is available from the Library of Congress

ISBN 0 7506 4983 6

For information on all Butterworth-Heinemann publications
visit our website at www.bh.com

Composition by Genesis Typesetting, Rochester, Kent
Printed and bound in Great Britain by MPG Books Ltd, Bodmin, Cornwall

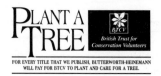

Contents

Contributors

Carl Backmän RGN
Senior Intensive Care Nurse, Department of Anaesthesia and Intensive Care, Vrinnevisjukhuset, Norrköping, Sweden

Kristine Carr RGN, DPSN, BA (hons) Health Studies, MSc Clinical Nursing
Nurse Consultant – Critical Care, ICU, Whiston Hospital, Prescot, Merseyside, UK

John Coakley MD, FRCP
Director of ICU, Intensive Care Unit, Homerton Hospital, London, UK

Charlie Granger FRCA
Consultant in Anaesthesia and Intensive Care, Intensive Care Unit, Royal Lancaster Infirmary, Lancaster, UK

Richard D. Griffiths BSc, MD, FRCP, ILTM
Reader in Medicine (Intensive Care), Intensive Care Research Group, Department of Medicine, University of Liverpool, Liverpool and ICU, Whiston Hospital, Prescot, Merseyside, UK

Christina Jones RGN, BSc (Biochem), BSc (Nursing), PhD
Research Fellow, Intensive Care Research Group, Intensive Care Unit, Whiston Hospital, Prescot, Merseyside and Department of Medicine, University of Liverpool, Liverpool, UK

Daniel D. Kennedy MB, FRCA
Consultant Anaesthetist, Royal London Hospital, Whitechapel, London, UK

Shelagh Platt RGN
Sister, Intensive Care Unit, Homerton Hospital, London, UK

Saxon Ridley MBBS, MD, FRCA
Consultant in Anaesthesia and Intensive Care, Norfolk and Norwich Acute NHS Trust, Norwich, UK

Clare Sharland BN, RGN
Intensive Care Follow Up Sister, General ICU, Southampton University Hospitals NHS Trust, Southampton, UK

Maire Shelly FRCA
Consultant in Intensive Care, Intensive Care Unit, Withington Hospital, Manchester, UK

Paul Skirrow BSc
Research Assistant, Department of Medicine, University of Liverpool, Liverpool, UK

Carolyn Temple BDS, MSc, DDPHRCS
Director of Community and Priority Services, Chester and Halton Community NHS Trust, Runcorn, UK

Jess Townsend RGN
Sister, Intensive Care Unit, Homerton Hospital, London, UK

Carl Waldmann FRCA
Director of Intensive Care, Intensive Care Unit, Royal Berkshire Hospital, Reading, UK

Duncan Young BM, DM, FRCA
Clinical Reader in Anaesthetics, Nuffield Department of Anaesthetics, Radcliffe Infirmary, Oxford, UK

Introduction – Why is ICU follow-up needed?

Richard D. Griffiths and Christina Jones

Background

The early years of intensive care medicine focused on what could be done and to whom. As great as the developments were, there were still many who considered intensive care as a 'service stop-over' with little concern for where the patients came from or where they were going. In the late 1970s and early 1980s attention became drawn, partly through spiralling costs, to being able to assess how ill patients were and to relate this to their ICU and hospital survival. This was very much an exercise in population description and survival outcome but resulted in the development of the illness severity measures we routinely use today. Unlike our neonatal colleagues who, from the start, have been preoccupied with the functional outcome of their infants, adult intensive care paid little heed to what happened to patients after they had left the unit except to count those who died. The neonatal specialists established elaborate follow-up programmes, but the usual practice following adult intensive care was for patients to be returned to their admitting speciality. This often meant that their follow-up was in terms of the admitting diagnosis and might not reflect upon the problems that developed as a consequence of their ICU stay.

A number of UK Intensive care units with physicians as a part of the team did follow-up a proportion of their medical admissions, notably Dr Alastair Short (Chelmsford) and Dr Steve Atherton (Whiston). In 1988, with their stimulation and in response to a request from the Kings Fund Panel (1989), a collaboration with the University of York (Centre for Health Economics) resulted in the first UK exploration of the costs and outcome from adult intensive care in terms of mortality and morbidity at 6 months (Shiell et al., 1990). Using quality of life measures, this preliminary study identified a significant degree of morbidity across a range of modalities and that, at 6 months, over two-fifths of patients still found that their health restricted their daily activities and one-fifth reported serious disability or distress. It also confirmed the futility of assessing survival and outcome at ICU discharge.

Over the last 20 years there have been many detailed questionnaire studies that examine whole intensive care populations or particular cohorts of patients. These have done much to show the relationship between such factors as pre-morbid health, age, illness severity and length of stay and outcome in terms of broad measures of function. Questionnaire follow-up will tell you a certain amount, but the choice of questionnaire used and the questions asked have to be guided by some knowledge of the anticipated problems. It is only through direct interview and physical examination that unexpected problems can surface.

Because the development of intensive care at Whiston hospital had always had physician involvement, the experience of Dr S T Atherton, who was seeing a proportion of ICU patients in his routine medical clinics, suggested that ICU patients had particular problems and a prolonged convalescence. In 1990, as part of a research programme, an ICU follow-up clinic was set up at Whiston Hospital. Through seeing patients on the wards a few days after intensive care and in an outpatient setting at 2 months and 6 months we were able to build a picture that demonstrated a core of problems, both physical and psychological, that characterized patients recovering from critical illness (Griffiths,1992). While some of these problems are closely related to particular diagnoses, others are far more generic in nature and reflect extremes of general illness severity and the challenges of a prolonged intensive care stay. Our early work used questionnaires to define the pre-morbid health status of our patients (Jones et al., 1993) and we related this to questionnaires applied in parallel to the clinic. However, we soon realized that questionnaires only gave the answer to the question you asked and not surprisingly were heavily influenced by pre-morbid health status, diagnosis and age as well as the ICU variables and patient perceptions. Furthermore, because we were dealing with patients of such wide ranges of pre-morbid health, age and primary diagnosis, the ability to interpret the data into information that could inform ICU care or help patients recover was extremely limited. Only recently, with data drawn from thousands of patients, has it proved possible to start to unravel some of the confounding variables, such as age (Hamel et al., 1999).

The doctors and nurses need ICU follow-up

As we met with patients and their relatives we realized that our questionnaire data were not going to help these patients. Furthermore, because the doctors they were seeing rarely dealt with patients who had been so ill or were primarily interested in only the original diagnosis, there were significant problems that were not being addressed. Is it necessary, however, that intensive care doctors or nurses be involved? Indeed, it has been suggested that the follow-up of ICU patients could be left to their general practitioner. The average GP will have little or no knowledge of what transpired and, having only a small number of patients who have had a stay in ICU, cannot be expected to know what problems they are likely to encounter. General practitioners are understandably skilled at post-hospital care but, after major surgery, this is done in partnership with the speciality so that the outcome of their actions is assessed. If intensive care is truly to develop as a speciality it has to understand the complete path of the illness process. This is the heart of the reason why the responsibility for intensive care follow-up must in part lie with the ICU doctors and nurses. The speciality needs to understand the outcome of its patients if it is to develop and improve the care of patients within intensive care. This process will inevitably identify problems after intensive care that can be solved in partnership with other specialities and the general practitioner. Leaving this responsibility to a broad range of specialities that have a variable understanding of intensive care is also unrealistic and will not lead to improvement in care. In many areas of medicine the primary pathology leads to disturbance in only one organ system and this is reflected in the development of organ-based specialities. Many of these specialists when pressed will admit to a limited continued experience of other system disorders. It is significant, therefore, that intensive care doctors and nurses who have developed the knowledge and skills to deal with multisystem disorders in the most severely ill ICU patients do have the expertise that can contribute to understanding the multisystem recovery that is required.

Research and development of our technologies and therapies in intensive care must call upon robust measures of outcome in both survival and morbidity terms. Outlining the common problems encountered by patients during their recovery and then designing studies that can test interventions to prevent problems or improve recovery is the only way forward. Our personal experience suggests that this can only be understood with involvement of a follow-up programme (Griffiths et al., 1997). This lack of insight may explain why there are still some commentators that believe it is not possible to use survival or morbidity outcome measures to test the effectiveness of therapies within intensive care.

Patients want ICU follow-up

Actually, at first, it is relatives who want the follow-up because, as will be discussed in later chapters, many patients do not recall that they have been in intensive care. Nevertheless, they still have problems and with 10 years of experience we can look back on full clinics and thankful patients as testimony to an unmet need. This alone cannot be justification unless we can show that the problems we identified needed to be treated or explained and that the new problems we described have led back to improved care within intensive care or afterwards. The soul of this book is about what we can do to help our patients and we hope starts to address this. Our goal must be patient well-being.

Society wants ICU follow-up

Society is now developing a new relationship with the medical profession that requires full understanding and agreement. *Perhaps the most compelling reason for patients to expect follow-up is for them to find out what was done to them while they were unable to give their consent.* The importance of patient follow-up has been recognized by the recent evaluation by the Audit Commission of UK critical care services (Audit Commission, 1999) which gave a high priority to follow-up services for all ICU patients. Similarly the UK government white paper, Comprehensive Critical Care (Department of Health, 2000), made it clear that all UK ICUs should be following-up their patients.

References

Audit Commission. *Critical to Success. The place of efficient and effective critical care services within the acute hospital.* Audit Commission, London: October 1999.

Department of Health. *Comprehensive Critical Care. A Review of Adult Critical Care Services.* HMSO, London: 2000.

Griffiths RD Development of normal indices of recovery from critical illness. In: *Intensive Care Britain 1992* (Rennie MJ, ed.). Greycoat Publishing, London: 1992, pp 134–7.

Griffiths RD, Jones C, Palmer TEA Six month outcome of critically-ill patients given glutamine supplemented parenteral nutrition. *Nutrition* 1997; **13**, 295–302.

Hamel MB, Davis RB, Teno JM *et al.* Older age, aggressiveness of care, and survival for seriously ill, hospitalized adults. SUPPORT Investigators. Study to understand prognoses and preferences for outcomes and risks of treatments. *Annals of Internal Medicine* 1999; **131**(10), 721–8.

Jones C, Hussey RM, Griffiths RD A tool to measure the change in health status of selected adult patients before and after intensive care. *Clinical Intensive Care* 1993; **4**, 160–5.

Kings Fund Panel Intensive care in the United Kingdom. *Anaesthesia* 1989; **44**, 428–31.

Shiell AM, Griffiths RD, Short AIK, Spiby J An evaluation of the costs and outcome of adult intensive care in two units in the UK. *Clinical Intensive Care* 1990; **1**, 256–62.

Immediate problems after ICU

Neuromuscular problems and physical weakness

Daniel D. Kennedy, John Coakley and
Richard D. Griffiths

Introduction

Muscle weakness is the most obvious and debilitating feature of recovery from critical illness. Within intensive care clinicians have recognized that muscle weakness may compromise recovery of patients, contributing to prolonged mechanical ventilation and all the risks of prolonged ICU stay. Subsequent hospital stay is prolonged and with the additional physiotherapy and rehabilitation, muscle weakness adds considerably to the cost of caring for these patients. Although our understanding of the contribution of the acquired neuromuscular disorders to the weakness associated with critical illness has improved considerably, currently these conditions cannot be predicted, prevented or treated effectively. The complexity of the critical care setting means that establishing a precise diagnosis can be difficult and the pathophysiology, aetiology and pathogenesis are still not well understood. Moreover, the pattern of onset, evolution and resolution of these disorders has not yet been clearly defined.

It was recognized for many years that intensive care patients developed significant muscle atrophy and subsequent weakness was attributed to catabolic muscle wasting. In the 1980s, however, evidence emerged of the development of acquired neuropathies in the critically ill patient – critical illness polyneuropathy (CIP) (Bolton et al., 1984), myopathies (Kupfer et al., 1987), or a combination of both (Op de Coul et al., 1985). Together these conditions account for the majority of lower motor neuron (LMN) lesions seen in ICU patients. Less commonly, there may be drug-induced neuropathies or generalized demyelination precipitated by infection. Although some patients will have disorders which may be associated with chronic neuropathy, such as diabetes, renal failure or cancer, if they are not known to have neuropathy before the onset of their critical illness, an acute neuropathy is unlikely to be a result of that disorder.

When muscular weakness is first noted in intensive care, it is often difficult to establish a cause for the problem. Clinical signs may be unreliable in the presence of sedative drugs and muscle relaxants, or where there is pre-existing cerebral dysfunction associated with sepsis or head injury. The possibility of central nervous system pathology (such as intracranial haemorrhage, infarction, infection) often needs to be excluded. This chapter, however, addresses those LMN lesions, neuromuscular transmission (NMT) defects and myopathies that befall ICU patients and their subsequent effect on recovery after intensive care.

Pathological changes in nerves during ICU

Critical illness polyneuropathy

The most commonly reported abnormality is critical illness polyneuropathy (CIP) which is characterized by axonal degeneration of motor nerves, that is loss of the central conducting part of the nerve. There is some evidence that the lesion in CIP is in the terminal motor axons, the nerve fibres nearest to the muscles (Schwartz *et al.*, 1997). Sensory nerves may also be affected either alone or in combination with motor nerve damage. It is unclear whether sensory nerve involvement is a result of the same process affecting motor nerves, other causes (such as entrapment or drug therapy) or a result of pre-existing neuropathy (such as diabetic or vitamin deficiency).

The precise aetiology of CIP has yet to be established, but it has variously been linked with sepsis, multiple organ failure (MOF), over feeding, hyperpyrexia, changes in osmolality, certain antibiotics and muscle relaxants. A common feature of studies in this area is that only those patients with obvious clinical weakness have been recruited, thereby selecting a group of long-stay, severely ill patients, most of whom will have had sepsis and organ-system failures at some time in their illness. In one study (Witt *et al.*, 1991), patients who had sepsis and MOF were studied prospectively and the only significant clinical correlation for patients who developed CIP was hyperglycaemia, hypoalbuminaemia and length of ICU stay. These associations are unlikely to be causative and probably reflect the presence of sepsis and severity of illness. CIP, however, has also been recorded in patients who do not fulfil conventional criteria for sepsis (Coakley *et al.*, 1993) and in those with only a single organ failure (Coakley *et al.*, 1992). Serum markers for sepsis, such as tumour necrosis factor, are no higher in patients with CIP compared to non-weak controls (Verheul *et al.*, 1994). This suggests that the aetiology is multifactorial, probably including many of the factors mentioned above. It has been suggested that there is a combined disturbance of both nerve and muscle that could account for the neuromuscular dysfunction complicating critical illness (Breuer, 1999). Table 1.1 gives some of the typical changes seen in nerve and muscle.

Table 1.1 Patterns of neurophysiological and muscle abnormality in 44 critically ill patients (Coakley *et al.*, 1998)

Group	N	(%)	Compound muscle action potential	Sensory action potential	Muscle biopsy
I	7	(16)	Normal	Normal	Normal (2) Diffuse fibre atrophy (1)
II	4	(9)	Normal	Reduced	Diffuse fibre atrophy (2) Type II fibre atrophy (1)
III	11	(25)	Reduced	Normal	Diffuse fibre atrophy (3) Neurogenic atrophy (2) Myopathy (3)
IV	19	(43)	Reduced	Reduced	Diffuse fibre atrophy (6) Neurogenic atrophy (1) Myopathy (3)
V	3	(7)	Not classified	Not classified	Myopathy (2)

Other neuropathies

Other neuropathies may coexist with CIP and may go unrecognized in the recovering patient. Diabetic patients commonly develop a distal, predominantly sensory neuropathy in a characteristic 'glove and stocking' distribution. Symptoms of numbness, paraesthesia and sometimes pain in the feet are associated with loss of vibration and position sense. Other isolated nerve palsies occur (mononeuritis), typically in the ulnar nerve that is exposed as it runs around the elbow and the common peroneal nerve as it passes around the outer aspect of the leg below the knee. Diabetic amyotrophy, a disorder that causes weakness and wasting of the quadriceps muscles, usually improves with better diabetic control and may go unrecognized in the wasted ICU patient.

Vitamin B deficiencies, common in alcoholics, may give rise to peripheral sensory neuropathies, presenting as numbness, pain and paraesthesia in the feet. Vitamin supplementation may improve these symptoms and prevent the development of megaloblastic anaemia but, more importantly, the very severe subacute combined degeneration of the spinal cord and consequent irreversible damage.

Following-up patients has allowed us to recognize likely entrapment neuropathies. Although the risk of pressure damage to peripheral nerves in ICU patients is quite widely appreciated it does still occur. Changes in nursing practice, such as prone ventilation, have brought out new problems. The nerves at particular risk are the common peroneal where it traverses the fibular head, the radial nerve in the spiral groove of the humerus, and the ulnar nerve in the ulnar groove around the elbow. The result may be a foot or wrist-drop and weakness in the hand. Persistent common peroneal nerve palsy has been reported long after resolution of coexisting CIP (Hund *et al.*, 1996), and we have also observed similar problems in long-stay ICU patients many years after recovery from the acute illness. It is possible that this is a long-term result of CIP, but clearly could also be a result of entrapment.

Peripheral neuropathies have long been associated with administration of drugs. Drugs commonly used on ICU that are known to cause neuropathies include phenytoin, metronidazole, amiodarone and hydralazine. Patients with cancer may have mixed, sensorimotor (involving both motor and sensory nerves) neuropathies associated with weakness and wasting of the proximal limb muscles around the upper arm and shoulder and thigh and pelvis.

Demyelinating disease

Guillain-Barre syndrome is a particular long-term problem both within ICU and for recovery afterwards. It is characterized by widespread demyelination (loss of the covering around nerves that permits fast nerve conduction) and usually presents to the ICU with respiratory weakness. It may rarely present as a result of ICU-acquired infection. Demyelination may be distinguished from axonal degeneration by analysis of cerebrospinal fluid, which typically shows increased protein content without any other abnormality. Electrophysiological testing in such cases will reveal reduced nerve conduction velocities and prolonged distal latencies. There is a rare axonal variant of Guillain-Barre syndrome (Feasby *et al.*, 1986) which may be difficult to distinguish from CIP initially, but has a different aetiology and prognosis. In contrast with the good recovery over a year seen in young patients with demyelinating GB, we have seen GB patients with axonal damage who have very slow and only partial recovery that takes many years.

Neuromuscular junction and myasthenia

Prolonged neuromuscular blockade, although a rare cause of long-term weakness in ICU patients, may exacerbate disuse atrophy and secondarily lead to weakness following ICU. The theoretical possibility of damage to the motor end-plate from prolonged use of neuromuscular blocking agents (NMBA) has led to histological examination of the neuromuscular junction (NMJ) in some patients. The most commonly reported finding is an increase in the number of acetylcholine receptors (Dodson *et al.*, 1995). Other work has demonstrated features of enlargement and regeneration of muscle end-plates (Wokke *et al.*, 1988). However, a myasthenia-like syndrome (where the muscle fatigues on repetitive use) is not seen, nor any abnormality detected by neurophysiological studies.

Patients with myasthenia gravis may require intensive care when bulbar or respiratory weakness is severe or following thymectomy. Therapy that produces optimal respiratory function may under- or over-treat other muscle groups, and some facial, bulbar or limb weakness may persist after discharge from the ICU. Weakness in these patients is exacerbated by repetitive or sustained effort, producing ptosis, diplopia, and impairment of speech and swallowing. Limb weakness, when it occurs, is usually symmetrical and typically affects proximal or upper limb muscle groups. When muscle weakness develops in a previously stable patient, it should be categorized as either a myasthenic (due to the disease) or cholinergic (due to the treatment) crisis, and treated accordingly. The two conditions may be differentiated by the response to edrophonium, which is positive in myasthenic weakness.

Pathological changes in muscle during ICU

Muscle wasting

Muscle wasting will occur as a result of any peripheral neuropathy. There is evidence that muscle tissue and its microvasculature is involved in the pathophysiological processes of multiple organ failure (Helliwell *et al.*, 1998b). In critical illness there are the added features of immobility, malnutrition and the catabolic effects of the stress response to surgery, trauma and sepsis. The administration of corticosteroids and neuromuscular blocking agents to asthmatic patients needing mechanical ventilation is associated with the development of muscle damage. Corticosteroids alone are known to produce proximal muscle weakness and wasting after acute or chronic administration. Muscle weakness has been related to the total dose of muscle relaxant used (Douglass *et al.*, 1992) and to the duration of use when administered by infusion (Behbehani *et al.*, 1999). Myopathies are also described, however, in non-asthmatic patients and in the absence of corticosteroids and neuromuscular blocking agents. CIP and acquired myopathies are probably superimposed on a background of disuse atrophy, malnutrition and the catabolic effects of serious illness. The severity of illness itself (as judged by the presence of sepsis and MOF) seems to be associated with the development of these problems and the use of corticosteroids and neuromuscular blocking agents may precipitate or more likely exacerbate this myopathy in some patients. The relative contribution of neuropathy and myopathy to weakness in these patients remains unclear, but it seems highly unlikely that either occurs in isolation.

Lean tissue and skeletal muscle wasting

Ever since Cuthbertson (1930), protein breakdown has been recognized as a metabolic response to injury. As severity of injury and sepsis increases then loss of lean (muscle) tissue predominates. Confirmation of this in the critically ill patient has come from detailed whole body composition studies made possible by siting the measuring equipment adjacent to an intensive care unit. Sequential studies in severely septic patients with peritonitis over 23 days (Plank *et al.*, 1998) showed that patients initially gained about 12 l of body water in the first couple of days of resuscitation but this was then steadily lost. Patients lost about 1.21 kg of protein (13%), of which two-thirds of this protein loss came from skeletal muscle in the first 10 days alone, but later more was lost from the viscera. The total loss of skeletal muscle mass was estimated to be 3 kg. These losses of lean body mass (whole body water and protein) that range from 0.5 to 1.0% loss per day is far greater than that due to bed rest alone. It should be remembered that the losses of protein are going on in the context of apparent full provision of nutritional support and are not related to starvation. The almost obligatory nature of this protein loss from skeletal muscle has been recognized for many years, but it is the rapidity and extent of the catabolic muscle wasting in the critically ill that has not been fully appreciated. Muscle biopsy studies on ICU show losses of muscle protein approaching 2% per day (Gamrin *et al.*, 1997). Histological changes in muscle are evident within the first few days with necrosis being an unusual late event (Helliwell *et al.*, 1991). In the very severely ill patient, serial biopsies taken in the first 10 days show that the mean daily decrease in the fibre area is 4% in type 2 fibres (faster contracting) but also 3% for the slower type 1 fibres that are more used for posture (Helliwell *et al.*, 1998a). It should be realized that the biopsies having the largest fibres show the greatest atrophy. The muscles show early loss in the contractile myosin filaments with relative preservation of actin and the structural proteins such as desmin. The systems involved in protein breakdown, such as lysosomal and ubiquitin proteolysis, are increased. Electron microscopy and immunostaining suggest that the individual myosin filaments break apart before undergoing extensive proteolysis. The early loss of myosin with the retention of the structural proteins may imply that these fibres have the potential to recover.

Inactivity and muscle pathology

A feature common to severely ill patients is the marked inactivity of their muscles. In healthy subjects immobilization of a limb results in muscle atrophy. In part this can be ameliorated by activity or letting the muscle undergo electrically stimulated contractions (Gibson *et al.*, 1988). Workers from France suggested that muscle wasting in the severely ill could be reduced by similar means (Bouletreau *et al.*, 1986). What is not clear is whether it is the muscle contraction *per se* or the forces and stresses induced in the muscle that prevent atrophy. Studies where normal volunteers lay for 30 days in head down tilt as a pseudo-weightlessness model to imitate a reduction in gravitational stress has shown a number of structural changes in human skeletal muscle which imitate some of the features seen in the critically ill (Hikida *et al.*, 1989).

Passive stretching of muscle

The question whether passive stretching of muscle alone could alter the structural and biochemical processes in the critically ill patient has been examined (Griffiths *et al.*, 1995). One leg was passively stretched and the other leg acted as the control for all the general metabolic and nutritional influences. To exclude the effect of voluntary contractile activity the patients received neuromuscular blocking agents so that any forces on the muscle were strictly passive and not influenced either by central drive or stretch reflex activation. There was preservation of muscle architecture with reduced protein loss and less fibre atrophy. However, this was not by a mechanism involving stimulation of protein synthesis (as measured by ribosomal analysis) implying instead that the proteolytic activity was reduced. The striking preservation of the architectural structure of the muscle goes along with the concept of reducing proteolysis. From a clinical perspective the passive stretch study underlines the importance of preventing immobility and that, so far as the recovery of skeletal muscle is concerned, every effort must be taken to re-establish mobility (with load and stress on the muscle) as soon as possible.

Consequences of neuromuscular weakness after ICU

The functional consequences of muscle loss only become apparent as the patient starts to recover and has to breathe for him- or herself and is able to mobilize. The diaphragm and the other skeletal muscles of the respiratory system are not protected from the process of muscle loss, in keeping with that seen in malnutrition (Arora *et al.*, 1982). Recent work, however, shows that despite a 35–50% decline in respiratory and skeletal muscle function, there is less loss initially of cardiac mass or function in critically ill patients over the first 3 weeks, once cardiovascular stability has been established (Hill *et al.*, 1997). This is consistent with the sustained increased cardiac output usually observed. This is reassuring for many patients since exercise can therefore safely be encouraged. However, there are limited data beyond this period and anecdotal experience in severe burns trauma has shown dilatational cardiomyopathies occurring 6–8 weeks following injury.

The challenges faced by patients with global weakness are obvious. It is with lesser degrees of weakness or less obvious weakness that problems arise. The problems of eating, chewing and swallowing are discussed in Chapter 5 (Nutrition). However, upper limb wasting can be so profound that self-feeding can be prohibitively tiring. The ability to recover adequate cough power may take weeks since it requires a combination of respiratory muscle power, glottic coordination and sufficiently compliant lungs able to take a large breath. A combined sensory disturbance, especially if it compromises position sense, also presents a challenge to limited muscle power.

Case study

The following case illustrates the time scales of recovery.

A 31-year-old woman was admitted to the Accident & Emergency Department with a 10-day history of increasing shortness of breath. She was treated with nebulized bronchodilators, systemic steroids and antibiotics, but became increasingly dyspnoeic, suffered a cardiorespiratory arrest and aspirated stomach contents. After successful resuscitation she was admitted to the intensive care unit for mechanical ventilation and treatment of bronchoconstriction, aspiration pneumonitis and sepsis. A pregnancy test was positive but the fetus was spontaneously aborted. On day seven, sedative agents were withdrawn and ventilatory support was rapidly weaned over the following 48 h. It became apparent, however, that although eye-opening and nodding her head to command, she was tetraplegic, with diminished tone and reflexes in all limbs. An EEG and CT scan of her brain were normal, and a lumbar puncture yielded normal CSF. By now fully alert and cooperative, she reported severe blurring of vision, but had no other symptoms of sensory involvement. Further assessment revealed marked impairment of swallowing and cough and gag reflexes. On day 20, she was extubated and had no further respiratory difficulty, though severe dysarthria became apparent.

An EMG on day 21 showed characteristic signs of a critical illness myopathy and subsequent MRI scans of her brain and cervical cord were normal.

While on ICU and on discharge to a medical ward, she had daily physiotherapy for her chest, limbs, speech and swallowing. Daily follow-up revealed gradual improvement in limb muscle strength, speech and swallowing.

By day 30 (from ICU admission) she could raise her arms to head level and her cough and gag reflexes and swallow were considered strong enough to allow oral feeding. The dysarthria also slowly improved. Ophthalmic assessment revealed healthy eyes and eye movements, suggesting cortical damage as the cause of her visual impairment, but this also improved over time. At outpatient follow-up 2 weeks later, she had made further progress, scoring MRC power grade 4 out of 5 in all four limbs, was able to stand alone and to walk a short distance with assistance. She was speaking and eating normally, and her visual acuity was continuing to improve.

The rate of recovery in this patient compared favourably with that reported elsewhere for older patients diagnosed with CIP. Although cranial nerve or bulbar involvement did not feature, limb weakness was often profound after discharge from ICU. The time taken to walking unassisted varied from 2 to 4 months and many patients had residual neurological deficits up to 1 year later.

Assessment of neuromuscular problems after ICU

Neurological and functional assessment on the ward or in the clinic following ICU must take into account the problems the patient had and therefore likely complications the patient will sustain and their length of ICU stay. Follow-up evidence confirms that the length of stay on ICU (and days of ventilation) is the most important predictor of major physical mobility problems following intensive care. Indeed the physical aids that patients needed at 8 weeks following ICU was closely related to their length of ICU stay (Jones and Griffiths, 2000).

Clouding of consciousness, confusion and impaired cognitive function are not uncommon and will confound clinical examination on the ward. Once the oedema that collected on the ICU has subsided, the extent of muscle wasting can be determined and muscle power correctly referenced to available muscle bulk. Coexisting joint stiffness, which is relatively common, may limit this assessment, however. While intention tremor is not uncommon in our elderly patients it is rare to see other abnormal movements. History taking is important as patients are more likely to express sensory deficits through difficulty with handling small objects than can be shown on formal clinical testing, although electrophysiological abnormalities persist. While the predominant neuropathic features are distal, the muscle wasting, although global, is grossly manifested by proximal weakness of the hips or shoulders. Therefore, the most useful clinical assessments are those of body movement, rising from bed or chair, standing and walking. Balance is important to maintain confidence. Even in the absence of obvious neurological impairment, profound muscle wasting results in weakness of the postural muscles crucial for rescue when stumbling. It is for this reason that a most common complaint is difficulty walking over rough ground. The provision of a stick, especially in windy conditions can be of help. Similarly, they must be warned when they go home that while they may have recovered sufficient strength to climb the stairs they may lack the strength for a confident and controlled descent. Alternatively, they may only have sufficient strength to climb the stairs once in the day, making a stair assessment prior to hospital discharge of little practical use.

Therapy of neuromuscular problems after ICU

Physical therapy with occupational therapy is the mainstay of fostering recovery following neuromuscular difficulties and an approach to exercise will be discussed in Chapter 11 (Rehabilitation). The key, however, is recognizing the extent and severity of the weakness these patients have. As is discussed later many of the patients lacking any recall of their ICU experience fail to realize how weak they are while they are in hospital surrounded by nurses and physiotherapists. They have falsely high expectations of their ability. Often it is only when they fall or go home that the extent of their weakness is apparent. It is therefore important that relatives are made aware of the issues and difficulties and the time scales involved in recovery.

Although at 2 months sensory problems may be present, very few ICU patients remain troubled by this at 6 months and they are usually of secondary importance to the patient compared with any motor disability. Since exercise is fundamental to rebuilding wasted muscle, other clinical conditions need to be optimized to foster mobility. Treatment of heart failure, angina, asthma or joint disease must be complementary. Similarly, psychological problems, especially those that affect adequate sleep, must be adequately treated.

Conclusion

The muscle wasting in the critically ill has many causes that include inadequate nutrition, neuropathic and myopathic processes, problems secondary to sepsis and intense cytokine stimulation, neurohumoral disturbances, drug therapy, all combined with inactivity. That muscle serves an important physiological role should not be underestimated. From a clinical standpoint the critically ill patient must get better and move to restore lost muscle. Particularly with an increasing ageing population, the critically ill patient has an outcome clock ticking away that is related to their starting mass of muscle. The more muscle you have the greater the size of the insult and the longer you can suffer before a critical muscle reserve is reached.

The longer the ICU stay the more profound will be the muscle wasting, myopathy and polyneuropathy and this will prolong convalescence (Leijten *et al.*, 1995). Only in the severest axonopathy, however, is prognosis guarded. Otherwise the outlook is more promising, based upon personal experience over the last 10 years of following the recovery of patients who have stayed a long time on ICU. It is reassuring that if the patient survives to leave hospital there is considerable return of nerve and muscle function, although it may take more than a year if the weakness was profound.

References

Arora NS, Rochester DF Respiratory muscle strength and maximum voluntary ventilation in undernourished patients. *American Review of Respiratory Disease* 1982; **126**, 5–8.

Behbehani NA, Al-Mane F, D'yachkova Y, Pare P, Fitzgerald JM Myopathy following mechanical ventilation for acute severe asthma. The role of muscle relaxants and corticosteroids. *Chest* 1999; **115**, 1627–31.

Bolton CF, Gilbert JJ, Hahn AF, Sibbald WJ Polyneuropathy in critically ill patients. *Journal of Neurology, Neurosurgery and Psychiatry* 1984; **47**, 1223–31.

Bouletreau P, Patricot MC, Saudin F, Guiraud M, Mathian B. Effets des stimulations musculaires intermittentes sur le catabolisme musculaire des malades immobilises en reanimation. *Annales Francaises d'Anesthesie et de Reanimation* 1986; **5**(4), 376–80.

Breuer AC Critical illness polyneuropathy. An outdated concept. *Muscle and Nerve* 1999; **22**, 422–4.

Coakley JH, Nagendran K, Ormerod IEC, Ferguson CN, Hinds CJ. Prolonged neurogenic weakness in patients requiring mechanical ventilation for acute airflow limitation. *Chest* 1992; **101**, 1413–16.

Coakley JH, Nagendran K, Honavar M, Hinds CJ Preliminary observations on the neuromuscular abnormalities in patients with organ failure and sepsis. *Intensive Care Medicine* 1993; **19**, 323–8.

Coakley JH, Nagendran K, Yarwood GD, Honavar M, Hinds CJ. Patterns of neurophysiological abnormality in prolonged critical illness. *Intensive Care Medicine* 1998; **24**, 801–7.

Cuthbertson DP The disturbance of metabolism produced by bony and non-bony injury with notes on certain abnormal conditions of bone. *Biochemical Journal* 1930; **24**, 1244–63.

Dodson BA, Kelly BJ, Braswell LM, Cohen NH Changes in acetylcholine receptor number in muscle from critically ill patients receiving muscle relaxants: an investigation of the molecular mechanism of prolonged paralysis. *Critical Care Medicine* 1995; **23**, 815–21.

Douglass JA, Tuxen DV, Horne M *et al.* Myopathy in severe asthma. *American Review of Respiratory Disease* 1992; **146**, 517–19.

Feasby TE, Gilbert JJ, Brown WF *et al.* An acute axonal form of Guillain-Barre polyneuropathy. *Brain* 1986; **109**, 1115–26.

Gamrin L, Andersson K, Hultman E, Nilsson E, Essen P, Wernerman J Longitudinal changes of biochemical parameters in muscle during critical illness. *Metabolism* 1997; **46**, 756–62.

Gibson JNA, Smith K, Rennie MJ Prevention of disuse atrophy by means of electrical stimulation: maintenance of protein synthesis. *Lancet* 1988; **ii**, 767–70.

Griffiths RD, Palmer TEA, Helliwell T, Maclennan P, Macmillan RR Effect of passive stretching on the wasting of muscle in the critically ill. *Nutrition* 1995; **11**, 428–32.

Helliwell TR, Coakley JH, Wagenmakers AJM *et al.* Necrotizing myopathy in critically ill patients. *Journal of Pathology* 1991; **164**, 307–14.

Helliwell TR, Wilkinson A, Griffiths RD, McClelland P, Palmer TEA, Bone JM Muscle fibre atrophy in critically ill patients is associated with the loss of myosin filaments and the presence of lysosomal enzymes and ubiquitin. *Neuropathology and Applied Neurobiology* 1998a; **24**, 507–17.

Helliwell TR, Wilkinson A, Griffiths RD, Palmer TEA, McClelland P, Bone JM. Microvascular endothelial activation in the skeletal muscles of patients with multiple organ failure. *Journal of Neurological Sciences* 1998b; **154**, 26–34.

Hikida RS, Gollnick PD, Dudley GA, Covertino VA, Buchanan P Structural and metabolic characteristics of human skeletal muscle following 30 days of simulated microgravity. *Aviation, Space, Environmental Medicine* 1989; **60**, 664–70.

Hill AA, Plank LD, Finn PJ *et al.* Massive nitrogen loss in critical surgical illness. Effect on cardiac mass and function. *Annals of Surgery* 1997; **226**, 191–7.

Hund EF, Fogel W, Krieger D, DeGeorgia M, Hacke W Critical Illness polyneuropathy: clinical findings and outcomes of a frequent cause of neuromuscular weaning failure. *Critical Care Medicine* 1996; **24**(8), 1328–33.

Jones C, Griffiths RD Indentifying post intensive care patients who may need physical rehabilitation. *Clinical Intensive Care* 2000; **11**, 35–8.

Kupfer Y, Okrent DJ, Twersky RA, Tessler S Disuse atrophy in a ventilated patient with status asthmaticus receiving neuromuscular blockade. *Critical Care Medicine* 1987; **15**, 795–6.

Leijten FS, Harinck-de Weerd JE, Poortvliet DC, de Weerd AW The role of polyneuropathy in motor convalescence after prolonged mechanical ventilation. *Journal of the American Medical Association* 1995; **274**, 1221–5.

Op de Coul AAW, Lambregts PCLA, Koeman J, van Puyenbroek MJE, Ter Laak HJ, Gabreels-Festen AAWM Neuromuscular complications in patients given pancuronium bromide during artificial ventilation. *Clinical Neurology and Neurosurgery* 1985; **87**, 17–22.

Plank LD, Connolly AB, Hill GL Sequential changes in the metabolic response in severely septic patients during the first 23 days after the onset of peritonitis. *Annals of Surgery* 1998; **228**, 146–58.

Schwartz J, Planck J, Briegel J, Straube A Single-fibre electromyography, nerve conduction studies and conventional electromyography in patients with CIP: evidence for a lesion of terminal motor axons. *Muscle and Nerve* 1997; **20**, 696–701.

Verheul GAM, de Jongh-Leuvenick J, Op de Coul AAW, van Landeghem AAJ, van Puyenbroek MJE Tumour necrosis factor and interleukin-6 in CIP. *Clinical Neurology and Neurosurgery* 1994; **96**, 300–4.

Witt NJ, Zochodne DW, Bolton CF *et al.* Peripheral nerve function in sepsis and multiple organ failure. *Chest* 1991; **99**, 176–84.

Wokke JHJ, Jennekens FGI, van den Oord CJM, Veldman H, van Gijn J Histological investigations of muscle atrophy and endplates in two critically ill patients with generalised weakness. *Journal of Neurological Science* 1988; **88**, 95–106.

Acute psychological problems

Christina Jones

Introduction

Over the last 10 years the awareness of acute psychological problems following critical illness has been growing. The importance of understanding the link between what we do in ICU, for example in weaning from sedation and acute psychological problems, is paramount. Our actions in ICU have an impact on the patients' well-being and, while the balance is always in favour of aiding survival, there has to come a point at which we must also try to achieve the best physical and psychological outcome we can.

This chapter will give an overview of the research so far, will be illustrated with examples of real patients' stories and also examine strategies that can be used to prevent problems developing.

Some historical background

The Whiston Hospital Intensive care (ICU) outpatient clinic has been in existence since 1990 and some clear problems have emerged that affect many patients recovering from critical illness regardless of admitting diagnosis. Patients coming to clinic at 2 months post-ICU feel the need to go through their time in the unit in some detail. This is because the majority of patients do not remember being in ICU and so do not have any first hand knowledge of what has happened to them. Indeed, they may not appreciate how ill they have been. Patients consequently find it hard to understand the slowness of their recovery and can become irritable, depressed, with a feeling of hopelessness as time goes on. Often they feel they are not recovering as quickly as they should. For many patients, the realization about the severity of the illness does not sink in until they go home and find they cannot do the things they want to do. In addition, the lack of memory for the period of critical illness, coupled with vivid memories of nightmares, hallucinations or paranoid delusions, may be a possible contributor towards psychological morbidity during the recovery phase of critical illness (Jones *et al.*, 2000a).

The immediate psychological effects of critical illness and the intensive care unit (ICU) environment on patients are well recognized and anxiety, depression, hallucinations, sleep disorders and confusion have all been widely reported. In addition, a link has been postulated between the abnormal environment in ICU, with the lack of a clear night or day and continuous noise from monitors and alarms on infusion pumps, and the development of so-called 'ICU psychosis', resulting in hallucinations and psychotic behaviour.

Amnesia for factual events in ICU

Why amnesia following critical illness is important

Perhaps the key factor that divides ICU patients from many other seriously ill patients is the amnesia experienced for the time in ICU. This lack of recall may extend to include events prior to admission to hospital in about 40% of patients (Jones *et al.*, 2000b). Other patient groups may be left with similar physical problems but at least have a clear mental picture of how this happened. A direct consequence for ICU patients is a medically unrealistic expectation of the speed of recovery. It is unfortunate that the prevailing view among many healthcare professionals is that it is helpful that patients do not remember their stay in ICU, but this means that the patients cannot understand why they are so debilitated (Griffiths *et al.*, 1996). In addition, patients are often considerably distressed by physical changes resulting from the critical illness, such as taste changes or loss, poor appetite, lethargy or severe weight loss resulting in gross changes in body image. Over the time in ICU patients lose weight, often dramatically, but they do not see themselves in a mirror; it can cause devastating distress when patients go to the ward and finally see themselves for the first time (see patient story 1).

Other physical changes, such as hair loss, finger nail ridges and skin changes, e.g. dry, flaky skin, which are all indicators of the severity of illness they have undergone, even when seemingly minor, worry patients when they do not have any explanation for their presence.

Patient story 1

One patient was admitted with complications following a routine oesophagogastrectomy. He stayed on the ICU for 2 months but did not remember his time there. When he was finally discharged to

> the ward he was wheeled to the bathroom for a wash and saw his face in the mirror for the first time in 2 months. He was stunned; the face that looked back at him was not his own but that of a stranger, gaunt and terribly pale.

The whole process of going to the ward and home after critical illness can be traumatic. Patients' families have ambiguous feelings about their discharge to the wards and later home. The shortage or lack of step down care in many hospitals and the clear lack of follow through to the community leaves the patient and the family feeling, rightly or wrongly, abandoned. Even when families are told in advance and prepared for the move to the wards, these feelings are still there. The intense anxiety that those relatives feel while patients are in ICU (Jones and Griffiths, 1995) carries over to ward and home when patients are discharged, so that they feel the constant need to protect the patient. Unfortunately, patients often find this attention smothering and this can result in arguments. The differing experiences of the time in ICU lead to conflict as the patient often does not understand how ill they have been and think the family is overreacting (see patient story 2).

Patient story 2

> One wife would not let her husband lock the toilet door just in case he collapsed and she could not get to him. His response was annoyance; he said he had always locked the door and did not want to be interrupted by his young grandchildren.

Where the patient is an older teenager/young adult they complain about the loss of freedom. Parents in this situation find it difficult to allow the young person to make their own mistakes about how much rest they take and what to do or not do (see patient story 3).

Patient story 3

> One mother found it very difficult to stop herself from telling her son to phone her every hour when he first started going out on his own. For his part, although he had been told what had happened to him, he had no memory for the time in ICU and pushed himself too much and got desperately tired. He knew his mum was right about not overdoing it but still resented being told.

What factors in the ICU stay contribute to amnesia?

Severe illness as a cause of fragmentary memories and amnesia

Acute confusional states have long been noted to accompany febrile illness, particularly prior to the advent of antibiotics. Delirium develops over a short period of time, usually hours to days, and tends to fluctuate during the course of the day and affects memory, resulting in a dense amnesia for the period of the confusion. Islands of memory can remain and coincide with fluctuations in the patient's consciousness level. The incidence of pure delirium in critically ill patients is simply unknown and is likely to prove difficult to recognize, let alone quantify. However, it is likely that some of the amnesia experienced by critically ill patients can be attributed to delirium.

Delirium also causes profound disturbance to the sleep cycle. Slow wave sleep and rapid eye movement (REM) sleep are both important in consolidating memories (Stickgold, 1998). Sleep deprivation has been shown to be common in ICU patients (Hilton, 1976), with decreased or absence of stages 2, 3, 4 (slow wave) and REM sleep (Gazendam et al., 2000). So the consolidation of memories is likely to be poor in ICU patients simply because of sleep deprivation.

Therapeutic drugs affecting memory

Many of the therapeutic drugs, including sedative drugs and opiates, used in the ICU can cause problems with memory. Much of the literature on the effects of drugs on consciousness is from short-term use in the field of anaesthetics, where the specific aim is to produce a period of unawareness for the duration of the operative manipulation. Propofol, when used in anaesthetic doses in theatre, has been shown to cause amnesia for events leading up to the operation in 34% of patients, complete amnesia for the duration of the anaesthetic and amnesia for a time after in 4% of patients.

Most patients in ICU will only receive initial propofol doses of 0.3–4 mg/kg/h, which compares to 4–12 mg/kg/h for maintenance of full anaesthesia. However, continuous infusions for prolonged periods result in high tissue concentrations (Heffner, 2000). A small dosing study in normal volunteers found a strong negative correlation between recall for a list of words and blood levels of propofol. However, it is difficult to predict the effect of propofol on memory with ICU patients based on work in normal volunteers. The time scale of sedation is very different and the presence of organ failures and alterations in body compartment proportions may have effects on plasma levels of propofol. Midazolam has similar amnesic properties to propofol and also has addictive potential.

Anxiety, panic attacks, symptoms of acute post-traumatic stress disorder early in recovery

Anxiety, panic attacks and symptoms of acute post-traumatic stress disorder can occur very early in recovery. This can have profound effects on patients' recovery. There are likely to be a number of causative factors including withdrawal from sedative medication, vivid intrusive memories of delusions, as well as physical symptoms such as breathlessness.

Drug withdrawal

In the later stages of an ICU patient's stay as sedation is weaned off to allow the patient to breathe for themselves, withdrawal reactions can cause considerable distress. Withdrawal reactions on stopping benzodiazepines, such as midazolam, can develop very quickly. In ICU, tolerance to midazolam can be observed over a period of time, with infusion rates as high as 90 mg/h being reported. In addition, in critical illness, the metabolism of benzodiazepines by the body is very variable (Shelly *et al.*, 1987). The surprising finding in benzodiazepine withdrawal is the sheer length of the process, with acute withdrawal symptoms lasting 1–2 weeks and then gradually decreasing physical and psychological symptoms lasting many months. Acute withdrawal symptoms can result in paranoia, severe agitation and tachycardia, while longer-term symptoms can include severe anxiety and panic attacks. These symptoms may only manifest itself on the ward after discharge from ICU (see patient story 4).

Evidence suggests that a process of gradual withdrawal of benzodiazepines rather than the sudden cessation is more sensible in all patients who have had midazolam as an infusion for more than a couple of days (Eddleston and Littler, 1997).

Patient story 4

A patient with a long stay on ICU had proved very difficult to sedate and had required midazolam in large doses to keep him in bed. On discharge to the wards it was suggested in the discharge summary that he should be slowly weaned from his benzodiazepines. Unfortunately, the message was not received and within 24 h of discharge the patient was aggressive, paranoid and very shaky. On follow-up by the ICU staff the oversight was noted and a low dose infusion of benzodiazepine commenced. Within 1 h the patient was calmer and no longer paranoid. The infusion was slowly weaned off and replaced with a small dose of oral diazepam. Unfortunately, the patient could remember feeling that everyone was trying to kill him and remained bothered by this for some considerable time.

Delusional memories

Although ICU patients can have poor recall for external ICU events, they often can remember clearly delusional memories, such as hallucinations. Patients describe these memories as being very vivid, detailed and frightening. Flashbulb memories share these qualities and are frequently noted on learning the news of prominent events, for example the assassination of President John F. Kennedy (Brown and Kulik, 1977). Traumatic events frequently lead to formation of detailed 'flashbulb'-like memories. It is these memories that can be replayed in post-traumatic stress disorder (PTSD) (Krystal et al., 1995). It has been suggested that the importance and the emotional content of the traumatic event are the key factors (Conway, 1995). A frightening memory of a nurse trying to kill you without a balancing memory of the care received in ICU is likely to have great importance and emotional significance to that patient (see patient story 5).

Patient story 5

One patient was convinced that one of the male nurses had taken out a contract on him because the patient had insulted his wife. This was so real to him that he told his family and the nurses on the ward, who did not know how to respond. A psychiatric referral was made, but the psychiatrist felt rightly that it just reflected how ill the patient had been but did not say this to the patient. Only when the ICU follow-up took place was this delusion challenged. The nurse in the delusion, who could be identified from the patient's description, was asked to speak to the patient and tell him that this had not really happened. Gradually the patient began to understand and he lost the conviction that it was a real event.

It is likely even relatively unpleasant memories for real events during critical illness may give some protection from anxiety, panic attacks and PTSD-related symptoms following ICU discharge. This appears to be against a backdrop of recalling frightening delusional memories, such as paranoid delusions, where factual memories may give patients a better chance of recognizing that these memories (that is delusional) were not real (Jones et al., 2001). Challenging such firmly held beliefs is only likely to be successful if done early in the recovery period (Keller, 1988).

Clinical implications and early interventions

The presence of psychological problems suggests a need for early ward follow-up after ICU. A number of strategies can be used to help patients come to terms with memory gaps for the period in ICU. Going through the ICU notes with the patient and explaining what happened each day can be useful. Very few patients do not want to know and those with whom this is done report greater understanding of how ill they have been. Patient diaries, dealt with in detail in Chapter 12, serve the same purpose but probably have more impact because of the photographs and the lay language used. The important thing is returning the ownership of the illness experience to the patient.

Assessment of memories for ICU and anxiety at 2 weeks could identify those patients at risk of developing severe acute PTSD-related symptoms and early intervention instituted. Blanket counselling of all patients is inappropriate and possibly counterproductive (Macfarlane, 1988). Those patients continuing to experience PTSD-related symptoms at 1–3 months post-ICU should actively be treated, because of the high risk of developing chronic PTSD (Foa et al., 1999). At this early stage psychological interventions, such as exposure therapy and education about the normality of these reactions, are the recommended first-line treatments.

More research is needed to examine ways of reducing delusional memories of ICU and increasing factual recall. Simply reducing sedative drugs is unlikely to achieve that aim. Until we fully understand the memory processes taking place it is unlikely we will be able to reduce the delusional memories recalled by ICU patients.

References

Brown R, Kulik J Flashbulb memories. *Cognition* 1977; **5**, 73–99.

Conway, MA *Flashbulb Memories*. Lawrence Erlbaum Associates, Hove: 1995.

Eddleston J, Littler C Withdrawal of sedation in critically ill patients. *British Journal of Intensive Care* 1997; Nov, **7**(16), 216–22.

Foa EB, Davidson JRT, Frances A The expert consensus guideline series. Treatment of post traumatic stress disorder. *Journal of Clinical Psychiatry* 1999; **60** Suppl.16, 1–75.

Gazendam J, Freedman NS, Schwab RJ, Zwaveling JH Sleep disturbances in the intensive care unit. *Intensive Care Medicine* 2000; **26**(S3), S275.

Griffiths RD, Jones C, Macmillan RR Where is the harm in not knowing? Care after intensive care. *Clinical Intensive Care* 1996; **7**, 144–5.

Heffner JE A wake-up call in the intensive care unit. *New England Journal of Medicine* 2000; **342**(20), 1520–2.

Hilton BA Quantity and quality of patients' sleep and sleep-disturbing factors in a respiratory intensive care unit. *Journal of Advanced Nursing* 1976; **1**, 453–68.

Jones C, Griffiths RD Social support and anxiety levels in relatives of critically ill patients. *British Journal of Intensive Care* 1995; Feb, 44–7.

Jones C, Griffiths RD, Humphris GM Disturbed memory and amnesia related to Intensive Care. *Memory* 2000a; **8**(2), 79–94.

Jones C, Griffiths RD, Humphris GM, Skirrow P Memory, delusions and the development of acute post traumatic stress disorder-related symptoms after intensive care. *Critical Care Medicine* 2001; **29**(3), 573–80.

Jones C, Humphris GM, Griffiths RD Preliminary validation of the ICUM tool: a tool for assessing memory of the intensive care experience. *Clinical Intensive Care* 2000b; **11**(5), 251–5.

Keller K Research hypotheses for intervention with delusion-prone individuals. In: (Oltmans TF, Maher BA, eds) *Delusional Beliefs*. John Wiley & Sons, New York: 1988: pp 318–23.

Krystal JH, Bennett AL, Bremner JD, Southwick SM, Charney DS Towards a cognitive neuroscience of dissociation and altered memory function in post-traumatic stress disorder. In: (Friedman MJ, Charney DS, Deutch AY, eds) *Neurobiological and Clinical Consequences of Stress: From Normal Adaptation to PTSD*. Lippincott-Raven, Philadelphia, 1995: 239–68.

Macfarlane A The longitudinal course of post-traumatic morbidity: the range of outcomes and their predictors. *Journal of Nervous and Mental Disease* 1988; **176**(1), 30–9.

Shelly MP, Mendel L, Park GR Failure of critically ill patients to metabolise midazolam. *Anaesthesia* 1987; **42**, 619–26.

Stickgold R Sleep: off-line memory reprocessing. *Trends in Cognitive Sciences* 1998; **2**(12), 484–92.

Jo Coleman

Information Update Service

Butterworth-Heinemann

FREEPOST SCE 5435

Oxford

Oxon

OX2 8BR

UK

Keep up-to-date with the latest books in your field.

Visit our website and register now for our FREE e-mail update service, or join our mailing list and enter our monthly prize draw to win £100 worth of books. Just complete the form below and return it to us now! (FREEPOST if you are based in the UK)

www.bh.com

Please Complete In Block Capitals

Title of book you have purchased:...

....

Subject area of interest:..

Name:..

Job title:..

Business sector (if relevant):...

Street:...

Town:... County:..

Country:... Postcode:...

Email:...

Telephone:...

How would you prefer to be contacted: Post ☐   e-mail ☐   Both ☐

Signature:.. Date:..

☐ Please arrange for me to be kept informed of other books and information services on this and related subjects (✔ box if not required). This information is being collected on behalf of Reed Elsevier plc group and may be used to supply information about products by companies within the group.

FOR OFFICE USE ONLY

Butterworth-Heinemann,
a division of Reed Educational
& Professional Publishing Limited.
Registered office: 25 Victoria Street,
London SW1H 0EX.
Registered in England 3099304.
VAT number GB: 663 3472 30.

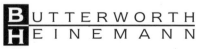

BUTTERWORTH HEINEMANN

A member of the Reed Elsevier plc group

Delusional memories of ICU

Paul Skirrow

> I remembered that I was supposed to deliver some stolen diamonds for the mob. Somehow I lost them . . . I don't know how . . . but I knew that they were going to get me when they found out! I thought that 'Chucky' – you know, that doll from the horror movie – was going to come and kill me!
>
> Later, when I realized where I was, I noticed that the nurses seemed constantly to be taking blood out of my arm. While nearly all of the other patients seemed to have gotten better and gone to the wards, I hadn't moved and didn't seem to be getting any better. Then it dawned on me – the nurses must be using my blood to cure everyone else. Once the blood ran out, they would have no use for me, so I knew I was done for. I thought that one of the doctors would come and slit my throat, and I was terrified.

The above description is based on the experiences of a 49-year-old male patient who spent a total of 50 days on the intensive care unit at Whiston Hospital. His experiences are typical of the remarkable experiences that patients often describe after a stay on intensive care – terrifying hallucinations and delusions of being kidnapped, incarcerated or even abducted by aliens (Waldmann and Gaine, 1996; Jones *et al.*, 2000). Similarly, the belief that doctors and nurses are secretly plotting to kill the patient is a recurring theme in the ICU follow-up clinic.

The importance of these frightening experiences in the ICU patient's physical and psychological recovery can sometimes be forgotten in follow-up. Although the knowledge that the *symptoms* of depression, anxiety, panic disorder and post-tramatic stress syndrome (PTSD) are common after ICU discharge has increased our ability to diagnose and refer patients with these difficulties, there remains little evidence as to what aspect of patients' ICU experience *causes* them to experience these problems. It is only now, after 10 years of follow-up that we are beginning to understand the profound effect that a patient's memory (or indeed, lack of it) from intensive care can have on their long-term recovery (Jones *et al.*, 2000).

In the introduction to this book, Richard Griffiths and Christina Jones argued convincingly that, although questionnaire-based studies are extremely useful in measuring specific problems after intensive care, it is only through a direct questioning that we can come to understand what constitutes a problem *for the patient*. For this reason, the present chapter seeks to describe one such problem, that of frightening hallucinations, delusions and nightmares from intensive care, which has consistently been highlighted by former patients as one of the most disturbing features of their ICU stay. The aim of the chapter is specifically to provide the ICU clinician with a general overview of these experiences, recognizing the importance of exploring hallucinatory and delusional memories and providing practical intervention skills.

What is a 'delusional' memory?

Psychologists and psychiatrists have tried for decades to answer this very question, with comparatively little success. Perhaps the most difficult aspect of delusions is their apparent 'falseness'. Although common sense dictates that the family of an ICU patient cannot actually have been replaced by aliens, proving to the patient that this is not the case is often easier said than done. Perhaps the best way to define a 'false' or 'delusional' memory is to allow the patient to do it for us. Often patients spontaneously talk about the strange dreams or hallucinations that they remember from being in intensive care.

- A dream, nightmare or hallucination experienced by the patient during their ICU stay.

Alternatively, patients can comment on the extreme confusion that they have experienced in intensive care, describing strange thoughts and experiences that, although very frightening at the time, they now know to be false. The individual described at the start of this chapter is a fine example of this. Although he was thoroughly convinced of their reality at the time, he later attributed these strange experiences to the medications he received while in ICU.

- A belief or memory of ICU that has been rejected as false by the patient.

Finally, on those rare occasions when patients continue to believe these experiences to be real (e.g. one man believed he had been on holiday for 1 month and refused to admit he had been in ICU), it generally falls to a consensus judgement to decide whether these experiences were real or imaginary. In the above case, for example, the man only conceded that he had been in ICU after his family cajoled him into speaking with the admitting consultant.

- A belief or memory of events in ICU that is not shared by medical staff or family members present during the patient's stay.

This is far from a satisfactory operational definition, since patients with fixed, persecutory delusions might easily interpret such a consensus as yet more evidence of the conspiracy! Some definition is required, though it is not unusual for patients to describe experiences that, although undoubtedly distorted, defy our best attempts to disprove them.

What kinds of experiences do patients describe?

In so far as any hallucinatory or delusional experience will undoubtedly be unpleasant for the patient, it seems evident that not all of the psychotic experiences will cause the patient to experience pathological distress after intensive care. With this in mind, the experiences of the ICU patient will typically fall into one of three broad categories, although it is important to note that patients often have experiences that fit into more than one of these categories.

- Benign hallucinatory experiences. Often patients describe bizarre hallucinations but have no negative feelings about them. For example, the patient may remember being on a cruise ship in the Pacific and, although this is far from the truth, will not necessarily find the experience particularly unpleasant.
- Hallucinations with a negative or delusional theme. Patients often describe hallucinations of gangsters or aliens (although this may be hard to distinguish from Capgras delusion, below) that have kidnapped or incarcerated them. Although not strictly delusional, these experiences can still be extremely frightening.
- 'Pure' delusions, i.e. without hallucinations. Perhaps the most frightening of experiences in ITU are those that are imbedded in reality, for example the nurse who tries to kill the patient with an injection in her foot, the doctor who decides who will live or die (both forms of persecutory or paranoid delusion), or the aliens doubles that have replaced the patient's family and friends ('Capgras' delusion).

Without doubt, it is those experiences that represent a form of threat or persecution that are the most upsetting for ICU patients. However, in a population where factual memories are few but depressive and anxious ruminations are high, it is important to explore the presence of *any* hallucinatory or delusional experience. In this respect, even the precise wording of a clinician's question can determine what experiences are revealed. General questions

Table 3.1 Examples of specific vs general questioning

General: *'What do you remember about intensive care?'*

Specific: *'Very often people tell us about all kinds of strange dreams or hallucinations from their time on intensive care. Sometimes they can even remember feeling that doctors and nurses on the ICU were actually trying to hurt them. Did you experience anything like that?'*

regarding a patient's memory of ICU can easily be misleading, suggesting only *factual* recall from intensive care. It is important, therefore, *always* to make a specific attempt to question about strange hallucinatory and delusional experiences and to stress that these experiences are extremely common. Table 3.1 provides some examples of questions that have been put to the recovering ICU patient. Note that the first example might be interpreted as meaning factual recall of intensive care, whereas the second is far more explicit.

Although the experiences of the intensive care patient are highly individual and no two will be precisely the same, there are a number of common themes that have emerged (see also Waldmann and Gaine, 1996). Themes of persecution or of personal danger seem particularly common in intensive care patients, as do themes of alien abduction and experimentation. Feelings of being trapped or incarcerated against the patient's will are also extremely common. Perhaps less extreme, however, are the common memories of being on a sea voyage, or of being on holiday in a foreign country. Again, the details of these experiences will vary from one individual to another, but the regularity with which these themes occur allows us to speculate as to their origin. For example, feelings of being on board a ship at sea may be seen to stem from the patient being nursed on the pressurized mattresses commonly used in intensive care.

Where do such strange hallucinatory and delusional experiences come from?

Much has been written on the actual causes of patients' hallucinations and delusions in intensive care. Many authors have suggested that they might be organic (e.g. Sitzman, 1993), psychological (e.g. Blacher, 1997) or, most popularly, environmental (e.g. Gelling, 1998). Each of these arguments has its individual merits, and while preventing ICU patients having these experiences at all must always be our ultimate aim, the current chapter is concerned with the aftercare of patients who have already been through intensive care and will not speculate upon their cause. However, many patients often attribute the cause of their hallucinations and delusions to the powerful medications used in intensive care or to part of the illness process itself. Certainly, in cases where patients have made accusations or shown inappropriate behaviour in intensive care, absolution of blame on the part of the patient is often a primary concern. In this respect, the knowledge that it is the majority of ICU patients that experience some hallucinatory or delusional episode can bring significant relief, as can some speculation on their cause. However, additional to this, many patients find it useful to understand just how they formed these strange ideas. For example, how do you come to believe that you are being forced to scrub the decks of an aircraft carrier when, in reality, you have been admitted to an ITU with severe pneumonia?

In order to understand how hallucinatory and delusional experiences are formed in ICU patients, it is useful to describe some of the psychological theories that relate hallucinations to normal perceptual experiences. In normal individuals, our perception of new objects or events is shaped, not only by what we see, but also by our previous understanding of the world in which we live. For example, when we see a man in a suit on a hospital ward, we are more likely to interpret this as meaning he is a doctor or a manager than a patient or a domestic because experience tells us that this is the most likely scenario. There is, therefore, an interaction between what we see and what we know about the world when we interpret new experiences. A similar process is believed to be at work when an individual has a hallucinatory experience. Somehow, however, these processes seem to have become distorted such that our interpretations of events appears to be shaped more by what we are expecting to see, than what is actually going on around us (Slade and Bentall, 1988).

Since hallucinations are shaped by both our environment and our own personal life experiences, these experiences are highly individual, but will often involve themes that are particularly important to the patient (Skirrow et al., unpublished data). For example, a woman who was extremely fond of her youngest granddaughter, came to believe that her granddaughter had, in fact, died and that her family were trying to hide it from her. Another man, who described a number of occasions on ICU when he was convinced that his house was about to burn down, later recalled that there had been a fire at his home a few weeks before he was admitted and that this had made him particularly upset.

Equally, the content of patients' hallucinations in intensive care is likely to be influenced by the environment around them (i.e. the ICU). Actual events in the intensive care can become twisted or distorted in meaning and patients often have extreme difficulty in separating their real memories from those they imagined. In this way, intensive care patients often take very real objects or events and transform them into something quite different. For example, one man described how he had come to think that the nurses' station in the middle of the unit was actually an elevator direct to Hell. Another woman described a belief that pair of burly male nurses washing the patient in the next bed were in fact female, blonde Scandinavians who were actually having intercourse with their patient.

Although identifying real ICU events that have become distorted, or experiences that represent real concerns felt by the patient at the time, some weeks after a patient has been discharged can be a nearly impossible task, this is not to say that it is not worth attempting. Through collaborating with the patient to place a more realistic interpretation on their bizarre or frightening experiences, the clinician provides an opportunity for the patient to understand their experiences and their implications in long-term recovery. Perhaps then, it is important to describe some of the longer-term effects of hallucinatory and delusional episodes on ICU and how they relate to the clinical picture in follow-up.

Why are these memories important in long-term follow-up?

Much has been made of ICU patients' inability to remember their time on intensive care, and this has been seen to be particularly detrimental to their physical and emotional recovery (see Chapter 2). Indeed, there seems little doubt that such a profound amnesia is an important factor in the development of acute anxiety and depression after intensive care. Perhaps more puzzling, however, is the apparently high incidence of post-traumatic stress disorder (a disorder characterized by intrusive 'flashbacks' of the traumatic event and an avoidance of reminders of the event) in this population (Schelling *et al.*, 1998). If patients have no memory for their time in ICU, how is it possible for them to experience intrusive 'flashbacks'?

Jones *et al.* (2001) have recently provided the answer to this intriguing question, with an innovative study of patients' memories from intensive care. By categorizing patients' memories according to whether they contained memories of frightening hallucinations or delusions and whether or not the patients had a *factual* recall of intensive care (as measured by a cued-recall task), Jones was able to show that it was the hallucinatory and delusional memories from intensive care that appeared to lead to the development of acute PTSD-related symptoms (Figure 3.1). Indeed, as Figure 3.1 clearly shows, it appears that a memory for factual events might actually *protect* against the development of acute PTSD. This is particularly interesting in light of the traditional view of hallucinations and delusions as 'dissociative' phenomena, that is a psychological defence, activated in order to escape from the real-life terrors (e.g. Abram, 1972).

The idea that a patient's memory for intensive care, whether factual or illusory, can influence their long-term psychological recovery is surely justification enough for the follow-up clinic. Certainly, the intensive care follow-up clinic remains a valuable 'safety net' in identifying patients with more general issues, such as depression or acute anxiety, which may be missed during routine visits to their general practitioner. However, the true importance of follow-up is apparent when we consider those physiological and psychological problems that are not only specific to ITU patients but also unlikely to be recognized by other healthcare workers. In this respect, the intensive care follow-up clinic will often represent the only opportunity for these patients to discuss such problems as the tethering of tracheostomy scars or, importantly, hallucinatory and delusional memories from intensive care. When we consider the high proportion of

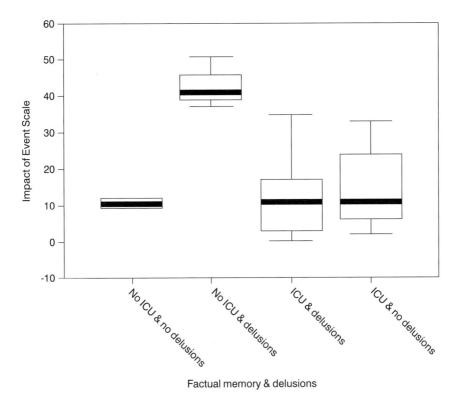

Factual memory & delusions

Figure 3.1 Memories of intensive care and acute PTSD-related symptoms (adapted from Jones *et al.*, 2001). No ICU = no recall of Intensive Care

intensive care patients who describe delusional experiences (Skirrow *et al.*, unpublished data, found an incidence of 88% in patients with a stay over 72 h) and the distress that these experiences can cause, it seems vital that follow-up should *always* address these issues.

Since patients will almost invariably realize that their memories are false after they have been discharged, and will often laugh and joke about their experiences, it has long been assumed that hallucinations and delusions cease to be a problem after discharge. In the same way that we comfort a child awaking from a nightmare, it has been assumed that simply knowing that 'it's not real' is enough to stop the memory from being frightening. Current research suggests that this is not always the case yet, for the same reasons, it may be difficult for a patient to admit distress caused by memories that they know not to be real.

There are, however, a significant minority of patients who will continue to believe their experiences, and particularly experiences of staff trying to kill them, to be real. It is for this reason that early ward-based interventions are vital in follow-up. Imagine a patient whose experience of intensive care included the belief that a doctor had tried to poison him while on intensive care. It does not take a great leap of imagination to suggest that he will be extremely wary of seeking medical help in the future, indeed, should he later receive an outpatient appointment to visit an intensive care physician he could hardly be blamed for not attending. For this very reason it seems clear that follow-up should, ideally, include both an early, ward-based intervention assessing patients' memories of ICU and a longer-term outpatient clinic to monitor their psychological impact.

How can follow-up help patients cope with their more disturbing experiences?

The present chapter has attempted to provide a general overview of the kinds of nightmares, dreams, hallucinations and delusions that patients often describe in intensive care follow-up. It also set out to provide insight into both the causes and the consequences of such disturbing experiences. Such an understanding, however, would have little value if it did not allow us to provide patients with better, more sympathetic follow-up. In summary, therefore, it is important to state explicitly the value of intensive care follow-up in helping patients to cope with their experiences. This is particularly important in three key areas:

1 Follow-up should provide an opportunity to talk about hallucinations and delusions. This is undoubtedly the most important role for follow-up in dealing with illusory memories from intensive care, since it may provide the patient's only opportunity to discuss these experiences without fear of social reprisal.
2 Follow-up should provide alternative explanations for unusual experiences.
3 Follow-up should allow for early interventions when necessary.

Still relatively little is known about the best ways to combat the adverse physical and psychological effects of a stay in intensive care, or indeed about their precise causes. However, it is becoming increasingly obvious that the presence of hallucinatory or delusional memories is particularly important in the development of long-term psychological ill health after intensive care. It is vital, therefore, that we continue to address the issue of illusory or false memories in the follow-up clinic.

References

Abram HS Psychotic reactions after cardiac surgery – a critical review. *Seminars in Psychiatry* 1972; **3**(1), 70–8.

Blacher RS The psychological and psychiatric consequences of the ICU stay. *European Journal of Anaesthesiology* 1997; **14**(Suppl. 15), 45–7.

Gelling L Causes of ICU psychosis: the environmental factors. *Nursing in Critical Care* 1998; **4**(1), 22–6.

Jones C, Griffiths RD, Humphris G Disturbed memory and amnesia related to intensive care. *Memory* 2000; **8**(2), 79–94.

Jones C, Griffiths RD, Humphris G, Skirrow PM Memory, delusions and the development of acute PTSD-related symptoms after intensive care. *Critical Care Medicine* 2001; **29**(3), 573–80.

Schelling G, Stoll C, Meier M *et al*. Health-related quality of life and post-traumatic stress disorder in survivors of acute respiratory distress syndrome. *Critical Care Medicine* 1998; **26**, 651–9.

Sitzman BT ICU psychosis: organic, psychosocial, or both? *The Psychiatric Forum* 1993; **16**(1), 33–9.

Skirrow PM, Jones C, Griffiths RDG, Kaney S (unpublished data). The impact of current media events on hallucinatory content in the ICU patient. Submitted *British Journal of Clinical Psychology 21/7/2000*.

Slade PD, Bentall P *Sensory Deception: A Scientific Analysis of Hallucinations*. Croom Helm Ltd, London: 1988.

Waldmann C, Gaine M The intensive care follow-up clinic. *Care of the Critically Ill* 1996; **12**(4), 118–21.

Part

2

After discharge from hospital

Sexual problems and their treatment

Carl Waldmann

Michel de Montaigne (1533–92)

Montaigne discussed sexuality in his first book of Essays. He knew a Gascon nobleman who, after failing to maintain an erection with a woman, fled home, cut off his penis, and sent it to the lady to 'atone for his offence.' Montaigne thought impotence was a very common experience, nothing to get too worried about, and blamed this extreme reaction on a lack of open discussion on the subject.

Introduction

There is no doubt that sex is an essential part of our complete physical and emotional well-being and recovery of this function is indicative of a good recovery from critical illness. Withdrawal of sexual intimacy because of fear of failure can damage relationships and have a profound detrimental effect on the well-being of couples.

In the Intensive Care Follow-Up Clinic at The Royal Berkshire Hospital, sexual dysfunction was found to be a common source of dissatisfaction for patients (Quinlan *et al.*, 1998). In 62 patients between 1996 and 1998, 26% reported sexual dysfunction at 2 months, 19% at 6 months and 16% (10 patients) at 1 year. Of these 10 patients, seven were male and three were female.

Even though sexual dysfunction is common following ICU, it may go unrecognized and untreated despite a major impact on a patient's quality of life. It may seem inappropriate to be concerned with a patient's sex-life when they have recovered from a life-threatening illness, but even though this may be a reasonable approach at 2 months post-ICU, it is less reasonable as time progresses. Very often sexual problems are not discussed because it is perceived to be embarrassing.

> *The genital activities of mankind are so natural, so necessary and so right: what have they done to make us never dare mention them without embarrassment and to exclude them from serious orderly conversation? We are not afraid to utter the words kill, thieve, or betray; but those others we only dare mutter through our teeth.* (Michel de Montaigne, 1991)

All too often sexual dysfunction is ascribed to psychological problems after ICU, but in our clinic there is no correlation between post-traumatic stress disorder (PTSD) and sexual dysfunction, which is at odds with the evidence of recovery following burns (De Rios *et al.*, 1997).

Incidence

The initial findings at our ICU Follow-Up Clinic prompted Quinlan *et al.*, 2001 to devise a questionnaire dealing specifically with sexual function post-intensive care, which was given to all patients attending (Figure 4.1). The findings from 1998 to 2000 were presented at the Riverside/ICS meeting in London in December 2000 (Quinlan *et al.*, 2001). Any patient scoring their sex-life as lower than before ICU was judged to have sexual dysfunction. Twenty-two out of 57 patients (39%) had sexual dysfunction. They described one or more of the following experiences:

- Nine patients described having no desire
- Eight patients had desire but 'nothing works'
- Ten patients were limited by shortness of breath or surgical disfigurement
- One patient and two partners were worried that sex may precipitate their illness
- In four patients sex-life had improved.

Of the 22 patients, nine were referred for psychosexual counselling or treatment and two were given sildenafil (Viagra) by their GP. Fifty per cent of patients declined help. Symptoms of PTSD were sought again and no link found with sexual dysfunction. In one patient referred for help a diagnosis of Peyrone's disease was made. In Peyrone's disease, gross deviation in the penis occurs when erect, making intercourse very difficult.

The word 'impotence' is used for males unable to maintain an erection, but female sexual dysfunction should not be ignored. From our Follow-Up Clinic, we refer men and women to psychosexual counselling, but men are referred to Andrology Clinic run by urologists.

Royal Berkshire and Battle NHS Trust

INTENSIVE CARE FOLLOW-UP CLINIC

This questionnaire has been designed to give us useful information. Some questions are of a personal nature, but we should be very grateful if you could answer them as honestly as possible. We do not wish to cause offence.

Private and confidential
SEXUAL DYSFUNCTION QUESTIONNAIRE

1)   Are you in a regular relationship?   Yes   ❑   No   ❑

2)   If yes, how long have you been in your relationship?   _____

3)   How would you describe your sex life in the year previous to admission?

1 = Poor ❑ 2 = Not very good ❑ 3 = Quite good ❑ 4 = Good ❑ 5 = Very good ❑

4)   How would you describe your sex life now?

1 = Poor ❑ 2 = Not very good ❑ 3 = Quite good ❑ 4 = Good ❑ 5 = Very good ❑

5) a.   Self-stimulation (masturbation) is a common and normal activity in adults.
       Was this a normal activity for you before intensive care?   Yes   ❑   No   ❑

   b.   If yes, have you been able to do so since?   Yes   ❑   No   ❑
       (Any comments?)

6)   If your sex life has altered since your admission, what is the change?

7)   If your sex life has altered since your admission, what do you think has caused the change? Please tick one or more:

   Physical changes due to the illness   ❑
   (Please explain)

   Everything works OK, but I no longer have the desire   ❑
   My partner is now worried about having sex   ❑
   I am frightened that sex may cause me to be ill   ❑
   Nothing works anymore, but I do have the desire   ❑
   I have a better sex life than before   ❑

8)   Are you satisfied with your present sex life?   Yes   ❑   No   ❑

9)   Is your partner satisfied with your present sex life?   Yes   ❑   No   ❑

10) Has your general relationship with your partner changed since your illness?
                                                               Yes   ❑   No   ❑

11) If so, in what way?

12) Please write any comments on how the Intensive Care Unit experience has affected your sexuality, sexual relationships and sexual performance.

13) Has any other health professional asked you about changes in your sex life since your illness; or warned you that you might experience problems?   Yes   ❑   No   ❑

   If so, who?

   Thank you very much for your help in completing this questionnaire.

If the questions have raised any issues that you would like to explore further please mention them to the doctor in the clinic or the nurse who collects the questionnaire, as we may well be able to offer you help.

Figure 4.1 Sexual dysfunction questionnaire

Male problems

Sexual dysfunction in men post-ICU is usually manifest as impotence, though occasionally we find patients who suffer premature ejaculation. Erectile dysfunction is defined as the persistent inability to achieve and maintain an erection sufficient for satisfactory sexual activity. It affects 100 million men world-wide. For men in the 40–70 year age group, 25% report moderate dysfunction. There are now UK management guidelines for erectile dysfunction (Ralph and McNicholas, 2000) put together for the Erectile Dysfunction Alliance. It has long been recognized that erectile problems may act as a marker for other common illnesses. If a patient can manage an erection at some stage, but not when having intercourse then a psychological problem is the most likely cause. Certain medications can cause problems (Table 4.1) and the presence of certain medical conditions make an organic cause more likely (Table 4.2).

Most erectile dysfunction is multifactorial and a combination of psychological and physical management methods may be needed.

Table 4.1 Medications

- Antihypertensives
- Diuretics
- Antidepressants (SSRI)
- Antipsychotics
- Hormones (oestrogen)
- Clofibrate
- Antiepileptics (phenytoin, carbamazepine)
- Anti-parkinson's (e.g. L-dopa)
- H_2-blockers

Table 4.2 Medical conditions

- Aortic aneurysm surgery
- Prostate surgery
- RTA involving pelvis
- Radiotherapy to the pelvis
- Smoking
- Alcohol/drug abuse
- Diabetes

Treatment

If hormone replacement is contemplated, prostate specific antigen assay, as well as rectal examination should both be performed. Psychosexual therapy may be successful in 50–80% of patients (Hartman, 1998). However, such a service is not available uniformly throughout the UK.

Medications

Viagra (oral sildenafil) improves erectile response in 50–88% of patients (Eardley, 1998). Sildenafil is rapidly absorbed with a short plasma half-life and works by selectively inhibiting phosphodiesterase (PDE5). This inhibition results in an increase in cGMP causing smooth muscle relaxation, vasodilation and restores erectile function.

One of the issues surrounding Viagra is the cost. Patients have to comply with certain criteria in order to obtain it through the NHS. Many patients are being asked to pay £4.25 per 25 mg tablet. It is our feeling that ex-ICU patients should be exempt from having to pay.

Alprostadil can be given by intracavernous injection (Figure 4.2) or transurethrally (Figure 4.3). The latter method has a 65% success rate (Padma-Nathan *et al.*, 1997).

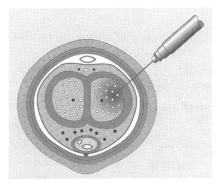 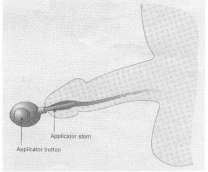

Figure 4.2 Intracavernous injection (reproduced from Wagner G, Saenz de Tejada I, 1998: 678–682 with kind permission of BMJ Publishing Group)

Figure 4.3 Transurethral application (reproduced from Wagner G, Saenz de Tejada I, 1998: 678–682 with kind permission of BMJ Publishing Group)

Vacuum devices

Vacuum (as depicted in the film 'The Full Monty') in conjunction with a ring fitted to the base of the penis results in engorgement of the penis (Figure 4.4). About 50% of users reported satisfaction with this device (Grahah *et al.*, 1998).

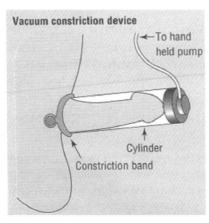

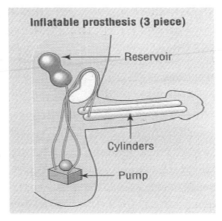

Fig 4.4 Vacuum device (reproduced from Wagner G, Saenz de Tejada I, 1998: 678–682 with kind permission of BMJ Publishing Group)

Figure 4.5 Penile prosthesis (reproduced from Wagner G, Saenz de Tejada I, 1998: 678–682 with kind permission of BMJ Publishing Group)

Penile prostheses

These should be considered for patients with organic causes of impotence, e.g. post-prostate removal, or when medical treatment or external devices fail. Technically the success rate is high (2.5% revision rate, 4.4% removal rate) (Evans, 1998) (Figure 4.5).

The cardiovascular patient

Because some patients recovering from a stay in critical care have cardiovascular problems, this must be taken into consideration when treating these patients for erectile dysfunction. Sexual activity is no more stressful to the heart than walking one mile in 20 minutes on the flat and the absolute cardiovascular risk of sexual activity is extremely low (Muller *et al.*, 1996).

The erectile dysfunction (ED) may be related to the drug treatment needed for their illness (see Table 4.1).

Patients with cardiovascular disease can be split into low, intermediate and high risk groups. The low risk group can be treated for ED without further cardiac assessment, but patients in the high risk group should be referred for cardiac assessment before providing ED treatment (Jackson *et al.*, 1999).

Obviously patients on warfarin cannot have intracavernous injection and Viagra should not be prescribed to patients on nitrates because of the risk of causing significant hypotension. Older patients should have a far lower dose of Viagra (25 mg) initially.

Female problems

Whereas in males sexual dysfunction can be easily diagnosed due to erectile problems, the situation in females is not so well defined. Female sexual dysfunction is age-related and may affect 30–50% of women (Laumann *et al.*, 1999).

Traditionally female sexual dysfunction has been considered a psychosomatic disorder; it cannot be overemphasized that organic causes must be excluded. Innervation involved in female stimulation is affected by dissection during pelvic surgery and can have a negative input on a woman's sexual health. Even a hysterectomy without oophorectomy can cause sexual dysfunction (Carlson, 1997). It is hoped that women are increasingly being offered nerve sparing pelvic procedures.

The first phase of female sexual function is desire and the next phase is that of excitement, evidenced by vaginal lubrication – corresponding to an erection in males. This lubrication is caused by increased blood flow throughout the pelvis. The third phase is known as the orgasmic platform, in which the clitoris elevates and finally, there is the resolution state in which blood flow virtually returns to normal.

The most common feature seen is hypoactive sexual desire (HSD) in which there are no fantasies for sexual activity. It is diagnosed when there is resulting interpersonal difficulty and marked distress as a result of the lack of interest in sex and it should not be due exclusively to the effects of drug abuse, diabetes or kidney failure. A 90-year-old frail woman or a single mother with two jobs and a full life may not have necessarily a great deal of sexual desire.

Sometimes one may see sexual aversion disorder in females who go to extreme lengths to avoid participating in sexual activity. Occasionally we find that these women have been subject to sexual abuse.

The second most common disorder is female sexual arousal disorder, where adequate lubrication cannot be maintained. In young women, the Pill or diabetes may account for this and result in a higher risk of developing vaginal infections, including candidiasis. Radiotherapy to the pelvis may also account for reduced lubrication; patients treated with antioestrogens for breast cancer may have similar problems, as do patients who have recently had pelvic surgery including hysterectomy.

Dyspareunia often has an organic cause and problems such as genital herpes need to be excluded.

Vaginismus may be the way sexual function is expressed and requires a good sexual therapist.

Management

Hypoactive desire

- Need to make correct diagnosis and exclude organic cause
- Give hormone supplements if hormone levels are low
- Bupropion hydrochloride sustained-release tablets
- Sexual psychotherapy

Sexual aversion

- Psychotherapy, counselling

Sexual arousal

- Treat underlying illness, e.g. diabetes to improve blood supply to vagina
- Topical oestrogens and oral supplements
- Topical testosterone
- Vitamin E suppositories (improves tissue tone in the vagina)
- KY jelly
- Patients on antidepressants, such as SSRI cannot have orgasms

Several companies are working on treatments for female sexual dysfunction. Zonagen (a US company) is developing Vasofem, which works by dilating blood vessels. Prostaglandin E cream may soon become available. An electrical clitoral suction device, which pulls blood into the area to help increase sensation and lubrication, is also being trialled.

The role of Viagra is as yet to be determined but it may work in females by increasing the blood supply to the vagina. Recent studies have demonstrated success with sildenafil in the treatment of sexual dysfunction due to ageing, menopause and secondary to the use of SSRI antidepressants (Goldstein and Berman, 1998).

Many people are convinced that as prostate surgery and diabetes can lead to erectile dysfunction in men, then hysterectomy, high blood pressure and diabetes can lead to circulatory problems and sexual dysfunction in women. In these situations Viagra may well help.

> The universal disobedience of this member which thrusts itself forward so inopportunely when we do not want it to, and which so inopportunely lets us down when we most need it. (Michel de Montaigne, 1991)

Discussion

It may be that locally there are inadequate facilities to treat both male and female sexual dysfunction. If the GP cannot help, The Impotence Association helps both men and women and also has a website, www.impotence.org.uk.

References

Carlson KJ Outcomes of hysterectomy. *Clinical Obstetrics and Gynaecology* 1997; **40**, 939–46.

De Rios MD, Novac A, Achauer BH Sexual function and the patient with burns. *Journal of Burn Care and Rehabilitation* 1997; **18**, 37–42.

Eardley I New oral therapies for the treatment of erectile dysfunction (review). *British Journal of Urology* 1998; **81**, 122–7.

Evans C The use of penile prostheses in the treatment of impotence. *British Journal of Urology* 1998; **59**, 1–8.

Goldstein I, Berman J Vasculogenic female sexual dysfunction. *International Journal of Impotence Research* 1998; **10**(2), 284–91.

Grahah P, Coling JP, Thissen AM Popularity of the vacuum erection device in male sexual dysfunction. *International Journal of Impotence Research* 1998; **10**(Suppl. 3), S6.

Hartman N The efficacy of psychosexual therapy for erectile dysfunction: a critical review of outcome studies. *International Journal of Impotence Research* 1998; **10**(Suppl. 3), S23.

Jackson G, Betteridge J, Dean J *et al.* A systematic approach to erectile dysfunction in the cardiovascular patient: a consensus statement. *International Journal of Clinical Practice* 1999; **53**, 445–51.

Laumann E, Paik A, Rosen R Sexual dysfunction in the United States prevalence and predictors. *Journal of the American Medical Association* 1999; **281**, 537–44.

de Montaigne Michel *Books 1, 2 & 3 The Complete Essays* (translated by MA Screech). Penguin, Harmondsworth: 1991.

Muller J E, Mittleman A, Maclure M *et al.* Triggering myocardial infarction by sexual activity. *Journal of the American Medical Association* 1996; **275**, 1405–40.

Padma-Nathan H, Hellstrom W J, Kauser FE *et al.* Treatment of men with erectile dysfunction with transurethral alprostadil. *New England Journal of Medicine* 1997; **336**, 1–7.

Quinlan J, Gager M, Fawcett D, Waldmann C Changes in sexual function after intensive care. *British Journal of Anaesthesia* 2001; **87**, 348.

Quinlan J, Waldmann C, Fawcett D Sexual dysfunction after intensive care. *British Journal of Anaesthesia* 1998; **81**, 809.

Ralph D, McNicholas T UK Management Guidelines for erectile dysfunction. *British Medical Journal* 2000; **321**, 499–503.

Wagner G, Saenz de Tijada I Update on male erectile dysfunction. *British Medical Journal* 1998; **316**, 678–82.

Nutrition after intensive care

Richard D. Griffiths

What is the nutrition challenge?

The period following intensive care is characterized by anabolism, remodelling, restoration and redistribution of body composition. This is not possible without an adequate nutrient delivery. The right foods are important, but the challenge is not in recognizing the need for adequate nutrition but in enabling the desire, delivery and ability to eat over the prolonged period of rehabilitation.

The extent of muscle wasting that occurs during a stay in intensive care is not always appreciated. As has been discussed in the earlier chapter on neuromuscular problems, a 3-week stay in ICU results in some 16% loss of total body protein. Such staggering losses of lean body mass (whole body water and protein) of almost 1% loss *per day* of illness is far greater than can be accounted for by the bed rest alone. Even the weightlessness of a long space flight produces losses of only one tenth of this. The greater part of the loss of lean body tissue occurs in the skeletal muscle, averaging about 2% loss per day. Forty days on the ICU would result in the loss of 4 kg of protein, most of which comes from the declining skeletal muscle pool. Since skeletal muscle accounts for about half of total body protein, it can be seen that muscle mass is suffering a 70–80% loss (Figure 5.1).

This vast protein store along with associated trace minerals and vitamins needs to be rebuilt. Increased protein intake is desirable but, for muscle growth, this must be linked directly to physical activity to promote efficient utilization and stimulation of protein synthesis. This will also take many months. ICU patients have undergone a period of negative nitrogen balance and usually also a period of negative energy balance. These are both however interrelated and studies of food restriction, inactivity and re-feeding show that food choice alters. Although total intake changes with the degree of exercise or inactivity, the proportion of

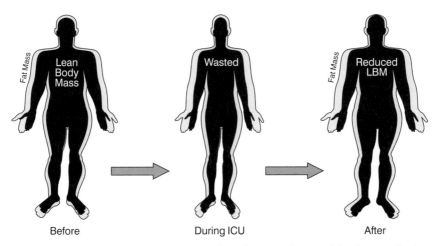

Figure 5.1 Muscle wasting is greater than fat mass loss and is also masked by tissue oedema. Fat mass re-accumulates faster than muscle mass

protein to energy usually changes little. The initial response to re-feeding is increased total intake through both energy and protein sensing mechanisms. However, the fat content of most western foods makes them intrinsically more palatable with a tendency to increased fat intake. Energy stores are more rapidly restored than the skeletal muscle protein and this will be exacerbated if exercise

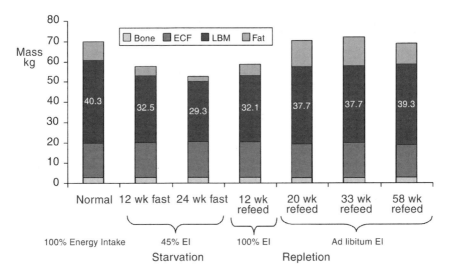

Figure 5.2 Normal volunteers undergoing starvation at 45% of energy intake, re-feeding at 100% energy intake and finally without energy intake restriction. Note more than a year is reached before full return of lean body mass. (Adapted from Keys A, Brozek J, Henschel A *et al. The Biology of Human Starvation.* University of Minnesota Press, Minneapolis, 1950).

tolerance is limited for other reasons such as respiratory insufficiency. Although during the first 6 months weight may be regained, this does not mean that the muscle mass (lean body mass) has been restored. The classic study by Keys *et al.* (1950) of body composition restoration following starvation shows this may take a year or more in some subjects (Figure 5.2).

As population demographics change we are recognizing type 2 diabetes more frequently in our elderly obese patients. Dietary management needs to be accommodated during recovery to avoid increased obesity relative to the reduced muscle mass and exacerbating the problem. For a number of patients an ICU admission discloses their type 2 diabetes.

During a severe illness many patients expand the extracellular fluid compartment with oedema. This often masks the extent of their muscle wasting. Following their illness it is not unusual for patients apparently to lose weight when they excrete this extra fluid as they start to recover.

Factors that limit intake

Once the patient has reached the general wards, it is a combination of desire, opportunity and physical problems that limit intake. Initially the desire or ability to eat may be limited by mood, taste changes, a small stomach, pain and fatigue. Delusions, depression and anxiety will all affect food desire. Neuroendocrine signalling may still be suppressed and extend the anorexic injury response. Concurrent medication may also be anorexic and adds to the misery these patients suffer. Taste changes are well described and these may make certain foods not just bland but even unpleasant. The availability of food is also a problem and depends on the family support around the patient, nursing and timing of food. Physical activity is a potent stimulator of increased food intake and for obvious reasons this may be absent.

The ability to eat depends upon a number of factors. Food delivery is affected by generalized muscle weakness that limits the ability of the patient to sit up, hold their head and use their arms to bring food to the mouth. Neuropathies alter touch, proprioception and fine motor control. Not so well appreciated is the difficulty of mouth opening with jaw joint stiffness and muscle weakness. Lost teeth or poorly fitting dentures affect chewing, but it is pharyngeal weakness and difficulty in the control of swallowing that is not appreciated. Pharyngeal weakness is usually part of generalized muscle wasting but can also occur in isolation following minor strokes.

With normal swallowing there is a voluntary stage when the tongue goes up and back against palate and swallowing receptors sense bolus. This is followed by the automatic pharyngeal stage (mediated via the medulla and pons). The soft palate closes off the posterior nares, the palatopharyngeal folds are pulled medially to guide the food. The vocal cords close, the larynx is pulled upwards and anteriorly by the neck muscles, and the epiglottis then swings backwards over the larynx. Finally, the upper end of oesophagus relaxes and the pharyngeal

Table 5.1 Some of the swallowing related problems

- Chewing weakness and bolus formation
- Impaired bolus sensation
- Feels unsafe to swallow or food sticks
- Regurgitates through nose (voluntary phase)
- Aspirates food (automatic phase)
- Splinting by tracheostomy
- Extrinsic sensation due to scars

muscle contracts with peristalsis from top down. This complex process requires good control and timing, particularly as it requires interruption of breathing. Sensory and motor deficits may upset the fine balance of the process. Recovering patients are more wary of swallowing and airway control, particularly if breathless or have been intubated for a long period or still have a tracheostomy. A cuffed tracheostomy tube may not only provide a physical pressure on the oesophagus but will splint the larynx and prevent it from rising during swallowing.

Table 5.1 lists some of the swallowing related problems.

Difficulty can be seen either by food being regurgitated, aspirated or by avoidance. A late complication of the new percutaneous tracheostomies is skin surface scar tethering and retraction. The small skin incision becomes fixed by fibrous tissue to the trachea. Every time the patient swallows they feel a pulling on the front of their chest as the larynx rises. A few patients find this sufficiently distressing so that surgical correction is required after one year.

The evidence that feed supplements are a benefit is varied. Their best utility appears linked with an exercise programme. A review of some 84 studies of 2570 patients, of which 45 were randomized, has shown that total energy intake can be increased. The benefits have been shown in certain populations of the elderly, notably those following hip fractures and chronic obstructive pulmonary disease and where the body mass index is $< 20 \, \text{kg/m}^2$. The improvements are seen in increased strength, fewer falls, and walking longer distances. Many of the complete feeds are found unpalatable by post-ICU patients and it is doubtful if additive feeds are nutritionally complete. However, where there is marked malnutrition and if food intake cannot be increased by other means there is benefit to be had by inter-meal supplements which have been shown not to reduce intake at meal times.

When I go home what foods should I choose?

Simple advice would be to take advantage of appetite and have small frequent meals. After a period of illness, especially with artificial nutrition, gastric volume distension may be reduced and a feeling of fullness develops with modest portion sizes. The act of eating, including chewing and swallowing, may be tiring and, if there is breathlessness, this extra work along with a feeling of abdominal fullness will add to the fatigue-inducing effect of a large meal. If gastrointestinal function has been seriously impaired it is worth avoiding large fatty meals. A broad balanced diet should be advocated. Warn of taste changes and that these will alter over the coming weeks or months. It is worth experimenting with different foods to find the most palatable as taste is central to food desire and consumption. Sometimes this can be improved by altering the food preparation method or adding a sauce or spice. Psychosocial factors will play an increasingly important role in nutrition during recovery. Food intake increases in proportion to the number of people eating and is reduced in the lonely and withdrawn. The diet of the recovering patient has to match a new lifestyle and often cessation of smoking. To foster an improved nutrition intake it is important to encourage eating as part of the social fabric of recovery. Avoid food intake as a solitary activity. Further, remind patients that food and eating are central to their recovery and well-being.

Patients should be encouraged to avoid excessive fat gain and obesity, as the extra weight is an unnecessary burden to weakened muscle. Prior eating and social habits will dictate the weight gain but fat re-accumulates more rapidly than skeletal muscle, particularly if exercise is lacking. Low protein intakes should be avoided, but there is no evidence that greater than normal protein intakes enhance lean body mass recovery. The importance of good food to recovery should be stressed and high quality foods, fresh fruit and vegetables encouraged. There is likely to be increased demand for antioxidants, trace minerals and vitamins during this period, although there is no evidence to support excessive additional supplementation. The advantage of specific substances to enhance muscle mass recovery and function is unproven, although they are fashionable in sports medicine. It is probably more important to link healthy eating with physical exercise to stimulate anabolic processes. This will encourage bone remineralization, muscle growth, fat redistribution, along with improved cardiovascular and pulmonary function and prevent obesity and type 2 diabetes.

Reference

Keys A, Brozek J, Henschel A *et al*. *The Biology of Human Starvation*. University of Minnesota Press, Minneapolis: 1950.

Physical and psychological recovery

Christina Jones and Richard D. Griffiths

Introduction

Specialist outpatient clinics after ICU have only a short history, but it has become clear that the physical and psychological problems patients encounter during their recovery can be profound. Key to the patients' physical recovery is the encouragement of physical activity and good nutrition. Aiding a patient's psychological recovery presents a much greater challenge, not least because our understanding of the process of recovery is in its infancy.

While this chapter will present an overview of the research so far, it will possibly pose more questions than answers about the strategies that can be used to prevent psychological problems developing.

Some historical background

The necessity for a prolonged period of convalescence after a serious illness, particularly in the days before antibiotics, has long been known. Florence Nightingale understood clearly the kind of physical weakness left by such illness and the strains it puts upon a patient during their recovery:

> Do not meet or overtake a patient who is moving about in order to speak to him, or to give him any message or letter. You might just as well give him a box on the ear. . . .You do not know the effort it is to a patient to remain standing for even a quarter of a minute to listen to you. (Nightingale, 1859).

With the advent of intensive care has come the ability to keep alive incredibly sick patients with major sepsis, resulting in catabolism of protein reserves in skeletal muscle. Such muscle losses happen rapidly but to rebuild require time, good nutrition and physical effort by the patient.

The history of research on the psychological effects of critical illness is much shorter and while the seriousness of the illness contributes to this, the memory problems that ICU patients report have a significant role to play.

Physical recovery post-ICU

For many patients, it is not until they go home that they first realize just how physically weak they are; commonly, climbing stairs is beyond them. Patients coming back to outpatient clinic at 8 weeks frequently report being surprised by how long it is taking them to get back to normal. Mobility at 2 months post-ICU is still very restricted, particularly outdoors. Of 148 patients coming to their 2-month outpatient appointment at Whiston Hospital, 44% either could not manage stairs or had difficulty climbing more than a few steps at a time (Jones and Griffiths, 2000); 29% were still using a wheelchair outside the house. Everyday activities we take for granted are major tasks for a convalescent ICU patient (see patient story 1).

Patient story 1

One patient described how she had offered to peel the potatoes for dinner while her sister was at work. She managed four potatoes in 40 minutes then had to have an hour's rest before peeling the other four.

As one would expect, the length of stay on ICU has an influence on the speed of physical recovery after discharge. The longer the stay the more likely patients are to need mobility aids at the 2-month clinic appointment (Table 6.1).

Similarly, as might be expected, age has an influence on recovery, with patients over the age of 50 years finding climbing stairs and walking outside much more effort (Figure 6.1).

The lack of a memory for the illness in ICU makes it hard for the patient to understand why they feel so awful. While staff and family may try to explain to the patient what has happened, the lack of a concrete memory means that patients often have unrealistic expectations of recovery, thinking of recovery in weeks, rather than months.

The majority of intensive care patients will not receive any physiotherapy once they are able to walk unaided in hospital. However, due to muscle loss

Table 6.1 Equipment used by patients to aid mobility at 8 weeks post-ICU, patients with ≤ median ICU stay compared to those with > median.

Equipment used	ICU stay ≤ 11 days (%) (n = 79)	ICU stay > 11 days (%) (n = 69)
Mobility outdoors		
Stick	5	17
Wheelchair	19	38
Zimmer	0	1
Stairs		
Unable/very difficult	38	51

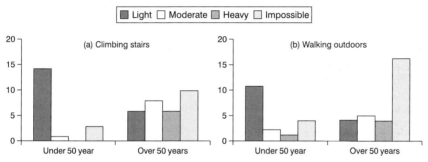

Figure 6.1 Perceived effort by patient while (a) climbing stairs and (b) walking outdoors by age (Jones and Griffiths, 2000)

and peripheral neuropathies their balance may be compromised and their ability to right themselves is very poor. Walking unaided outside in icy conditions or in a wind is potentially dangerous and frightening for the patient (see patient story 2).

Patient story 2

One patient said he constantly had at the back of his mind the worry about not having the strength to get home. This worry kept him from building up his activity as he always walked short distances that didn't really change over time. He eventually got himself out of this rut by buying a home exercise bicycle.

Table 6.2 Physical problems commonly seen after critical illness (Griffiths and Jones, 1999)

Recovering organ failure (e.g. lung, kidney, liver etc.)

Gross muscle wasting and weakness
- Including reduced cough power
- Pharyngeal weakness

Joint stiffness

Numbness, paraesthesia (peripheral neuropathy)

Taste changes resulting in favourite foods being unpalatable

Disturbances to sleep rhythm

Cardiac and circulatory decompensation
- Postural hypotension (autonomic neuropathy)
- Heart failure

Reduced pulmonary reserve
- Breathlessness on mild exertion
- Increased work of breathing

Iatrogenic
- Tracheal stenosis (e.g. repeated intubations)
- Tethering of skin to trachea (percutaneous tracheostomy)
- Nerve palsies (needle injuries)
- Scarring (needle and drain sites)

In addition, seemingly minor physical problems, such as hair loss, skin dryness, or fingernail ridges, which are common after critical illness, can be real causes of worry to the patients. Table 6.2 shows some of the problems commonly seen after critical illness.

Psychological recovery

Many of the physical factors that are likely to cause psychological distress in ICU patients are found in other groups of patients. Patients who have been through a critical illness are at risk of psychological problems because the nature of the illness is life-threatening, it may be of long duration and can leave conspicuous effects, such as gross weight loss and muscle wasting. However, the physical changes, coupled with the absence of recall for the illness, make ICU patients almost unique. The grief reaction that accompanies any new disability or functional loss is especially profound if the cause of the loss is sudden and can take 1–2 years to resolve (Kaiser Stearns, 1992). In addition, ICU survivors cannot always be assured that they will make a full recovery back to their pre-morbid health status. Recovery is very much dependent on the cause of the admission and the patients' pre-existing health problems, for instance, an ICU admission may be precipitated by an acute exacerbation of an already existing illness such as chronic lung disease.

Studies specifically looking at the longer-term psychological and psychosocial problems of critical illness identify patients avoiding company and showing less affection to their partners, which indicates a profile of social isolation and dependence on others (Benzer *et al.*, 1983). A large study involving 3655 patients found a high incidence of psychosocial dysfunction, particularly for patients

Table 6.3 Categories of psychological problems encountered after ICU (Jones *et al.*, 1998)

Categories	Examples	Consequences
Recurrent nightmares	Fear that people will think that they are going mad	Cannot face going to sleep May hide memories of bizarre and frightening nightmares
Agoraphobia	Panic attacks on going out alone	Stays at home Puts excessive demands on the relatives to accompany them everywhere
Panic and confusion	Panic attacks particularly when shopping or in crowds	Avoids shopping
Anger and conflict	Angry with themselves for not being back to normal Angry with relatives for trying to make them take it easy	Hostile to self Hostile to relatives
Fear of dying	Don't want to be alone in case they are taken ill again	Makes unreasonable demands for company
Depression	As time goes on and patients find they are not back to normal	Withdrawal Reluctant to ask for help with severe depression
Anxiety	As patients first realize how ill they have been	May delay seeking medical help
Guilt	For what they have put their family through while they were ill	Overcompensation to make amends to the family

between 30 and 50 years of age (Tian *et al.*, 1995). Patients experience considerable levels of depression, anxiety, irritability and social isolation (Jones *et al.*, 1994), with 33% of patients still very anxious at 6 months post-ICU (Jones *et al.*, 2001). Panic attacks are also common. Patients report feeling that the recovery phase of their critical illness is the most stressful period as they learned how ill and close to death they had been (Compton, 1991). Table 6.3 gives a list of some of the problems that patients encounter.

Memories of ICU and psychological distress post-ICU

The memories that patients have from their time on intensive care seem to have a considerable influence on later psychological distress. Those patients who recall delusional memories, such as paranoid delusions or hallucinations, at 2

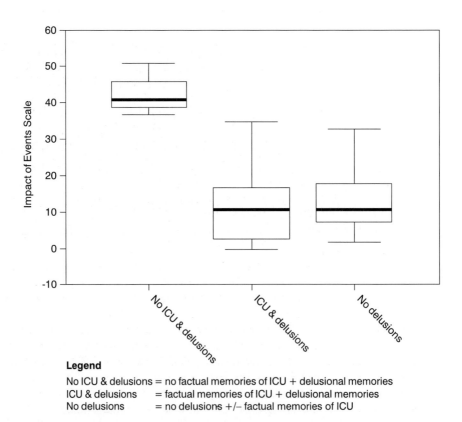

Legend

No ICU & delusions = no factual memories of ICU + delusional memories
ICU & delusions   = factual memories of ICU + delusional memories
No delusions   = no delusions +/– factual memories of ICU

Figure 6.2 Impact of Events Scale scores for the three patient group categories at 8 weeks according to factual or delusional memories at 2 weeks (Jones *et al.*, 2001)

weeks post-ICU but do not remember any factual events, are more anxious and depressed. In addition, these patients are more likely to develop acute post-traumatic stress disorder (PTSD)-related symptoms, such as intrusive thoughts and avoidance of reminders, as measured by the Impact of events scale (Jones *et al.*, 2001) (Figure 6.2).

Post-traumatic stress disorder

Post-traumatic stress disorder (PTSD) is a condition triggered by the experience of some horrific event out of the normal range of human experience. The stressor must be extreme, not just severe, and cause powerful subjective responses such as intense fear, helplessness and horror (Foa *et al.*, 1999). It is characterized by a range of symptoms, such as re-experiencing the event (flashbacks), avoidance of situations that remind one of the event, a numbed reaction and symptoms of increased arousal (see Table 6.4 for DSM-IV Criteria for PTSD, American Psychiatric Association, 1994).

If the symptoms have less than one month's duration they may be transient and self-limiting and would be diagnosed as an acute stress disorder (Foa *et al.*, 1999). Such a reaction can be regarded like grief, as a normal reaction to severe stress and has parallels with a grief reaction from a sudden bereavement. Generally everyone involved in a disaster will immediately experience some symptoms and behaviours related to severe stress. Twenty-eight symptoms have been identified that can occur in situations or events perceived as an immediate threat to life (Table 6.5). However, the presence of severe symptoms during this period is a risk factor for developing PTSD (Foa *et al.*, 1999).

Processing of the stressful event has been achieved when the individual can be reminded of the incident *without* distress. Using the same analogy, PTSD can be viewed as 'emotional indigestion' (Palmer, 1996).

If the duration of symptoms is 1–3 months then this would be diagnosed as acute PTSD and active treatment in this phase may reduce the high risk of developing chronic PTSD (Foa *et al.*, 1999). Once symptoms have been present for 3 months or longer then the diagnosis is chronic PTSD and longer, more aggressive treatment may be needed. It is also much more likely that co-morbid disorders, such as substance abuse, depression, panic disorders and generalized anxiety disorder will be present (Foa *et al.*, 1999). Alcoholism is common among sufferers of PTSD, as is caffeine and chocolate addiction (Turnbull, 1994). The tranquillizing effects of alcohol are frequently used as self-medication but can progress into alcohol dependence (Warsaw *et al.*, 1993). Opiate and benzodiaze-pine dependence are also reported in disaster victims, particularly if they needed hospitalizing for severe injuries (Sturgeon, 1993).

The incidence of PTSD in the general population as a whole is 1%, although the incidence is increased in high risk groups, e.g. among uninjured veterans of war 3.5% (Pitman *et al.*, 1989) and individuals injured in motor vehicle accidents 10% (Brom *et al.*, 1993). In a study of general ICU patients with an ICU stay of over 4 days, 15% were found to be suffering from PTSD at 1 year (Koshy *et al.*, 1997). A

Table 6.4 DSM-IV criteria for PTSD

The following six diagnostic criteria must be met for a diagnosis of PTSD

1 **The person has been exposed to a traumatic event in which both of the following were present:**
   - The person experienced, witnessed, or was confronted with an event or events involving actual or threatened death or serious injury, or a threat to the physical integrity of self or others.
   - The person's response involved intense fear, helplessness, or horror.

2 **The traumatic event continues to be re-experienced in one or more of the following ways:**
   - Recurrent and intrusive distressing recollections of the event, including images, thoughts, or perceptions.
   - Recurrent distressing dreams of the event.
   - Acting or feeling as if the traumatic event were recurring, including a sense of reliving the experience, illusions, hallucinations and dissociative flashbacks which can occur on awakening, when intoxicated, or at other times.
   - Intense psychological distress at exposure to internal or external cues that symbolize or resemble an aspect of the traumatic event.
   - Physiological reactivity on exposure to internal or external cues that symbolize or resemble an aspect of the traumatic event.

3 **Persistent avoidance of stimuli associated with the trauma and numbing of general responsiveness which was not present before the trauma, including three or more of the following:**
   - Efforts to avoid activities, places, or people that arouse recollections of the trauma.
   - Inability to recall an important aspect of the trauma.
   - Markedly diminished interest or participation in significant activities.
   - Feeling of detachment or estrangement from others.
   - Restricted range of affect, for example unable to have loving or angry feelings.
   - Sense of a foreshortened future, for example, does not expect to have a career, marriage, children, or a normal life span.

4 **Persistent symptoms of increased arousal, not present before the trauma, as indicated by two or more of the following:**
   - Difficulty falling or staying asleep.
   - Irritability or outbursts of anger.
   - Difficulty concentrating.
   - Hypervigilance.
   - Exaggerated startle response.

5 **Duration of the disturbance symptoms in 2, 3 and 4 for more than one month.**

6 **There is clinically significant distress or impairment in social, occupational, or other important areas of functioning.**

Table 6.5 Responses to trauma (Wilkinson and Vera, 1989)

Helplessness
Increased heart rate
Dyspnoea
Hyperventilation
Nausea
Vomiting
Extreme trembling or shaking
Excessive sweating
Dizziness
Feeling faint (light-headedness and unsteadiness)
Blurry vision
Hot flashes or flushing
Tingling sensations in the arms or hands (paraesthesia)
Diarrhoea
Urinary or faecal incontinence
Nervousness
Ringing in the ears
Outbursts of anger
Inability to remember recent events
Headaches
Pain
Restlessness
Hypersensitivity to sudden or rapidly changing stimuli (noise, light)
Sleep disturbances
Nightmares
Irritability
Difficulties in concentration
Feelings that familiar things are strange or unreal

---

second follow-up study of 80 ICU patients who survived adult respiratory distress syndrome showed an even higher rate of PTSD at 27.5% (Schelling *et al.*, 1998). In this study, those patients recalling a high number of adverse memories of ICU such as nightmares, pain, anxiety/panic or dyspnoea were much more likely to develop PTSD than those who did not. However, the patients in this study were asked about their recall of ICU anywhere from 6 months to 10 years post-discharge so the accuracy of the memories of some of the patients has to be called into question. Even very vivid traumatic memories can change over time (Conway, 1995). In addition, the patients only had to answer yes or no to the memory questions so the relationship of memories of anxiety, etc. to recalled nightmares is not clear. Jones *et al.* (2001) suggest that patients who had no factual memories of ICU but had some delusional memories, such as paranoid delusions, are more likely to develop acute PTSD-related symptoms (see Figure 6.2). Severe symptoms during the acute phase (< 3 months since the traumatic event) is associated with an increased risk of developing chronic PTSD.

Patient story 3

Patient 3 reported that she recalled that in ICU she thought that all her family had been replaced by aliens except for her mother. She remembered being frightened to go to sleep because the aliens wanted her body. She was very distressed by her memories of the delusion and complained of flashbacks. She subsequently refused to have further surgery she needed because she could not face having a general anaesthetic in case it all happened again.

It has been suggested that the quality of cognitive processing at the time of the traumatic event is important in the development of chronic PTSD. Those individuals who report feeling confusion and feeling overwhelmed as they experienced the traumatic situation are more likely to suffer from chronic PTSD (Ehlers and Clark, 2000). These individuals seem to lack perceptual processing of the traumatic situation, i.e. are unable to process the meaning in an organized way. They will instead concentrate on processing of the sensory impressions, termed data-driven processing, of the situation (Roediger, 1990). ICU patients may be predisposed to high levels of chronic PTSD. This may be because during the traumatic event, either due to the treatment instituted during the ICU stay or due to the critical illness, their ability to process information is likely to be compromised by a number of factors, such as critical illness, delirium, sleep deprivation, sedative drugs and opiates. They are likely to be unable to process the meaning of the events happening to them.

Recovery from trauma

The process of recovering from trauma has been broken down into three steps (Herman, 1992): attaining a sense of safety, remembering the details of the trauma and mourning the loss it has entailed, and finally re-establishing a normal life. The first step of attaining a sense of safety involves the individual learning ways of calming the increased arousal of the emotional circuits sufficiently to allow relearning. This can begin by the person simply recognizing that their agitation, hypervigilance and nightmares are all part of the symptoms of an acute stress reaction, making them less frightening. The next step in the healing process, of remembering the trauma and mourning the loss it has brought, involves reworking the story of the traumatic event. The memory is transformed to reduce the sense of the loss of safety. Where this occurs naturally there seems to be an inner clock that 'doses' people with intrusive memories so reliving the trauma, which is interspersed with long periods of weeks or months when they hardly remember anything (Horowitz, 1986). This seems to allow a spontaneous review of the trauma and relearning of the emotional response. In essence, debriefing is designed to facilitate this process soon after the trauma so that the memories do not become too overpowering. But, for those with established PTSD, recalling the trauma can lead to overwhelming fears, which interfere with relearning. They are unable to see the trauma as a time-limited event and instead have a 'sense of serious current threat' (Ehlers and Clark, 2000). This may result in safety behaviours to reduce the perceived likelihood of further dangers and can place severe limitations on socialization (Salkoviskis, 1996).

Mourning the loss the trauma brought allows the individual to start to look towards the future and rebuild a new life. This does not mean that there are no after-effects, but that the symptoms are at a manageable level. The memories can be revisited voluntarily like any other memory and then put aside. Joseph LeDoux (1992) puts it like this:

> *Once your emotional system learns something it seems you never let it go. What therapy does is teach you to control it. The propensity to act is suppressed, while your basic emotion about it remains in a subdued form* (p.192).

Southwick *et al.* (1995), as a result of a study of Gulf war combatants, suggest that the anxiety and hypervigilance are the first symptoms of possible PTSD and trigger unpleasant memories and thoughts. The rational mind is not involved in this process and it is possible that, if the anxiety and hyperarousal can be treated early, then the full PTSD syndrome will not develop. Alternatively the intrusive thoughts that are so characteristic of PTSD are actively suppressed and not worked through, increasing the frequency of unbidden thoughts and increasing anxiety (Wegner *et al.*, 1990). Interestingly the use of narrative writing by trauma victims has been shown to be beneficial but only if they express their emotions as well as telling the facts (Pennebaker and Beall, 1986). This is likely to be because writing helps to bring the trauma more fully into consciousness in a coherent story (Harper and Pennebaker, 1992).

Debriefing following a traumatic event has been used widely as an initial treatment and it is suggested that it is most effective undertaken as soon as possible after the traumatic event (Turnbull, 1994). One aspect of learning fear that has been well known for many years is the phenomenon of *incubation*, i.e. the delay between a trauma and the onset of psychological distress (Marks, 1987). It has been part of folklore that if you fall from a horse, then you should get back on to the horse as soon as possible, otherwise the fear of getting back on increases and may lead to the person never riding again. However, recent randomized controlled trials have found that, in some cases, a one-off session of early debriefing can increase the chance of individuals developing PTSD later, for example one study in fire-fighters found that debriefing counselling increased the danger of developing PTSD (Macfarlane, 1988). It is now suggested that interventions should be targeted at those showing the highest levels of acute traumatic symptoms. For this reason monitoring symptoms of PTSD and offering therapies, such as exposure therapy, anxiety management and psychoeducation about the normality of PTSD symptoms, to those at high risk of PTSD is now thought to be the most effective first line psychological intervention (Foa *et al.*, 1999).

Future work

As yet there has only been one randomized, controlled study looking at physical and psychological rehabilitation in ICU patients (see Chapter 14). Further studies are needed to verify the results of this study. In addition, further research is needed in a number of areas to reduce the psychological sequelae of critical illness, in particular the incidence of PTSD in ICU patients:

- studies are needed to understand the contribution that sedative and opiate drugs make to the recall of delusional memories from ICU
- a robust, well validated screening tool for PTSD is needed to identify patients at risk of developing chronic PTSD
- to understand the best way to help patients come to terms with their illness and their memories of ICU.

References

American Psychiatric Association *Diagnostic and Statistical Manual of Mental Disorders*, 4th edn. American Psychological Society, Washington, DC: 1994.

Benzer H, Mutz N, Pauser G Psychological sequelae of intensive care. *International Anaesthsiology Clinics, European Advances in Intensive Care* 1983; **21**(2), 169–81.

Brom D, Kleber RJ, Hofman MC Victims of traffic accidents: incidence and prevention of post traumatic stress disorder. *Journal of Clinical Psychology* 1993; **49**(2), 131–40.

Compton P Critical illness and intensive care: what it means to the client. *Critical Care Nurse* 1991; **11**(1), 50–6.

Conway MA *Flashbulb Memories*. Lawrence Erlbaum Associates, Hove: 1995, p. 116.

Ehlers A, Clark DM A cognitive model of posttraumatic stress disorder. *Behavioural Research and Therapy* 2000; **38**, 319–45.

Foa EB, Davidson JRT, Frances A The expert consensus guideline series – treatment of posttraumatic stress disorder. *The Journal of Clinical Psychiatry* 1999; **60**(suppl. 16), 1–75.

Griffiths RD, Jones C ABC of intensive care – Recovery from intensive care. *British Medical Journal* 1999; **319**, 427–9.

Harper KD, Pennebaker JW Overcoming traumatic memories. In: (Christianson, ed) *The Handbook of Emotion and Memory: Research and Theory*. Lawrence Erlbaum Associates, Hilldale, NJ: 1992, pp. 359–87.

Herman JL *Pathway to Recovery from Trauma. Trauma and Recovery*. Basic Books, New York: 1992.

Horowitz M *'Dosing' of Trauma: Stress Response Syndromes*. Jason Aronson, Northvale, New Jersey: 1986.

Jones C, Griffiths RD, Humphris GM, Skirrow P Memory, delusions and the development of acute post traumatic stress disorder-related symptoms after intensive care. *Critical Care Medicine* 2001; **29**(3), 573–80.

Jones C, Griffiths RD, Macmillan RR, Palmer TEA Psychological problems occurring after intensive care. *British Journal of Intensive Care* 1994; Feb, **4**(2), 46–53.

Jones C, Griffiths RD Identifying post intensive care patients who may need physical rehabilitation. *Clinical Intensive Care* 2000; **11**(1), 35–8.

Jones C, Griffiths RD, Humphris GH Disturbed memory and amnesia related to intensive care. *Memory* 2000; **8**(2), 79–94.

Jones C, Humphris GM, Griffiths RD Psychological morbidity following critical illness – the rationale for care after intensive care. *Clinical Intensive Care* 1998; **9**, 199–205.

Kaiser Stearns A *Living through Personal Crisis*. Sheldon Press, London: 1992.

Koshy G, Wilkinson A, Harmsworth A, Waldmann CS Intensive care unit followup program at a district general hospital. *Intensive Care Medicine* 1997; **23**(S1), S160.

LeDoux J Brain mechanisms of emotion and emotional learning. *Current Opinion in Neurobiology* 1992; **2**(2), 191–7.

Macfarlane A The longitudinal course of post-traumatic morbidity: the range of outcomes and their predictors. *Journal of Nervous and Mental Disease* 1988; **176**(1), 30–9.

Marks IM *Fears, Phobias and Rituals*. Oxford University Press, Oxford: 1987.

Nightingale F. *Notes on Nursing: What it is, and What it is not*. Harrison & Sons, London: 1859, p 29.

Palmer IP Practical aspects of post-traumatic stress reactions. *Presentation to the Injury Research Group*, Manchester 1–2 April 1996.

Pennebaker JW, Beall SK Confronting a traumatic event: Towards an understanding of inhibition and disease. *Journal of Abnormal Psychology* 1986; **95**, 274–81.

Pitman R, Altman B, Macklin M The prevalence of post-traumatic stress disorders in wounded Vietnam veterans. *American Journal of Psychiatry* 1989; **146**, 667–9.

Roediger HL Implicit memory: retention without remembering. *American Psychologist* 1990; **45**, 1043–56.

Salkovskis PM (ed.) The cognitive approach to anxiety: threat beliefs, safety-seeking and the special case of health anxiety and obsessions. In: *Frontiers of Cognitive Therapy*. Guildford, New York: 1996, pp 48–74.

Schelling G, Stoll C, Meier M *et al.* Health-related quality of life and posttraumatic stress disorder in survivors of adult respiratory distress syndrome. *Critical Care Medicine* 1998; **26**, 651–9.

Southwick SM, Morgan CA 3rd, Darnell A *et al.* Trauma-related symptoms in veterans of Operation Desert Storm: a 2-year follow-up. *American Journal of Psychiatry* 1995; **152**(8), 1150–5.

Sturgeon D Posttraumatic stress disorder. In: (Stanford SC, Salmon P, eds) *Stress – from Synapse to Syndrome*. Academic Press, London: 1993, pp 421–31.

Tian ZM, Reis MD Quality of life after intensive care with the sickness impact profile. *Intensive Care Medicine* 1995; **21**, 422–8.

Turnbull G Feeling the nightmare. *The Guardian* 1994; Tuesday February 22, 17.

Warsaw MG, Fierman E, Pratt L *et al.* Quality of life and dissociation in anxiety disorder patients with histories of trauma or PTSD. *American Journal of Psychiatry* 1993; **150**(10), 1512–16.

Wegner DM, Shortt JW, Blake AW, Page MS The suppression of exciting thoughts. *Journal of Personality and Social Psychology* 1990; **58**, 409–418.

Wilkinson CB, Vera B Clinical responses to disaster. In: (Gist R, Lubin B, eds) *Psychological Aspects of Disaster*. Wiley & Son, New York: 1989.

Aftercare programme – where, when, how and who?

Ward visits after intensive care discharge: why?

Kristine Carr

Introduction

For many people experience of an intensive care unit consists of the images portrayed by the popular media. The dimmed lights, hushed tones and subdued lighting bear little resemblance to the reality. Yet it is reality that confronts patients, relatives and friends when a profound illness necessitates an admission to a critical care area.

The long-term physical and psychological effects of a prolonged stay in intensive care are now well documented and recognized (Griffiths *et al.*, 1996; Mata *et al.*, 1996; Jones *et al.*, 1998; Jones and Griffiths, 2000). The critical care environment, the care delivery and even the illness itself are thought to contribute to the detrimental effects that a stay in an intensive care unit can have on some patients (Lloyd, 1993; Biley, 1994; Smith *et al.*, 1997; Jones and Griffiths, 2000). But, perhaps surprisingly, the experience may not always be a completely negative one. A small study of patients discharged from intensive care found that patients felt safeguarded while in the unit rather than stressed (Compton, 1991). Indeed, Saarmann (1993) states that 'the patient in a critical care unit often comes to see the nurse as a lifeline; a person carrying out lifesaving and life-sustaining measures'. It would come as no surprise that almost inadvertently those same nurses can also foster feelings of dependency in patients and their families at a time when they are feeling their most vulnerable and insecure.

Yet many patients will fortunately reach that point in their recovery from critical illness when discharge to a general ward is envisaged. For some, this may be viewed as a positive step on the continuing road to recovery and independence. Others may view the inevitable reduction in high-tech monitoring, nursing and medical attention, in addition to settling in an unfamiliar environment, as quite stressful. This phenomenon is often referred to as 'transfer anxiety' or 'relocation stress' (Saarmann, 1993; Cutler and Garnet, 1995; Whittaker and Ball, 2000). Although these rather simplistic terms fail to describe completely or explain the complex factors that can contribute to a patient's and his family's fear of discharge, they serve to highlight one problem area that may require active intervention post-discharge. But there are other, even more serious difficulties that the discharged patient can encounter and be required to overcome.

A number of factors may influence or even complicate the decision of when to discharge a patient from intensive care. In the ideal world this decision is reached when the multidisciplinary team is agreed that, clinically, the patient is ready to be managed less intensively. We know that the level of care and support available on the ward is generally significantly less than that in intensive care, so do not wish to discharge patients prematurely.

However, intensive care is an extremely expensive but limited resource, and one that we are constantly battling to use efficiently and effectively, particularly in times of increased need. Indeed, Bion (1995) proposes, rather strongly, that Britain's underfunding of intensive care probably results in avoidable illness and death. When the demand for intensive care beds is high, patients who might benefit from a slightly longer stay on the unit may have to be discharged to allow admission of a more critically ill person. Ideally, patients that may still be considered at risk of sudden deterioration would all be managed in step-down facilities or high-dependency units. Ridley (1998) suggests that such units can function as a means of bridging the gulf between the level of support available on the intensive care and general wards.

However, two major problems exist that may make this not a completely viable option. These facilities are also a limited resource and are not always available for all step-down intensive care patients. In addition, it is difficult to predict absolutely those patients at a high risk of deterioration who may benefit from a longer intensive care stay or transfer to a high-dependency unit (Rubins and Moskowitz, 1988). Nor is it easy to be completely sure that every patient discharged to the general ward is at low risk of a subsequent need for intensive care (Rubins and Moskowitz, 1988; Bone et al., 1995). What is very clear from all of the available evidence is that about 9–16% of discharges will require readmission to intensive care (Rubins and Moskowitz, 1988; Goldhill and Sumner, 1998). The major reason for readmission in 30–53% of patients was recurrence of their initial disease (Durbin and Kopel, 1993; Chen et al., 1998). Of those who developed a new complication, respiratory failure was found to be the major cause (Baigelman et al., 1983; Franklin and Jackson, 1983; Chen et al., 1993; Kirby and Durbin, 1996). But authors are all agreed that premature discharge could have contributed to the need for readmission in many cases. In particular, Goldfrad and Rowan (2000) identified a worrying and increasing trend towards premature discharge at night. These patients were found to fare significantly worse than those discharged during the day. In their view this only served to confirm that hospitals have insufficient intensive care beds to cope with an ever-increasing demand.

What could make night discharges particularly distressing for patients is that not only do they have their rest disturbed but also do not have time to adjust to the idea of leaving the security of the intensive care unit. In addition, because of the precipitous nature of such a discharge, medical and nursing handover of a patient who may still have significant physical and psychological morbidity, may be hurried and not as comprehensive as would normally be the case. It may not be possible to communicate with a representative of the team who will be assuming the care of that patient, as only on-call medical staff would be available. In addition, staffing levels on general wards at night are significantly lower than in daytime. Both medical and nursing staffs in these areas have a huge workload and limited time to give to an unexpected intensive care discharge, no matter how afraid and vulnerable that patient might be feeling. Nor does a night discharge give intensive care staff the opportunity to put in place the support from the multidisciplinary team that the patient may still require (i.e. respiratory physiotherapist, dietician, nurse specialists, etc.). There are many opportunities for communication breakdown to occur in this scenario with consequences for maintaining the quality and continuity of the patient's medical and nursing management.

But in all cases of readmission to intensive care, whatever the predisposing factor, these patients will remain hospitalized twice as long as survivors with uncomplicated courses and have a hospital mortality significantly higher than overall hospital mortality of all-comers to ICU (Rubins and Moskowitz 1988; Chen et al., 1998). This has overwhelming implications for the financial demands of providing this extended, unexpected medical and nursing care as well as the quality of life issues for these patients.

But even more worrying is that mortality on general wards after discharge from intensive care has been reported as varying from 6 to 16% (Rubins and Moskowitz, 1988; Bion, 1995) up to as high as 25%, including 50% with a low predicted mortality (Goldhill and Sumner, 1998). Without doubt death may have been inevitable for some of these patients, but Goldhill and Sumner (1998) state 'that care received after ICU may affect what will be recorded as an ICU death'. In effect, potential preventable ICU deaths are determined by events taking place outside of the ICU, a view substantiated by Wallis et al. (1997).

So do these patients still require our interest and intervention once they have been handed back into the care and responsibility of their referring medical team? The answer can only be a resounding yes! We owe more to these patients than simply to ensure that they have survived their critical illness. We have, in all probability spent thousands of pounds and hundreds of man-hours to achieve this successful outcome. Should all of these resources be wasted for want of, very often, some simple support and advice to ward medical and nursing staff post-discharge? Those who have cared for these patients in the intensive care unit are best placed to understand why they and their families behave as they do, particularly after a prolonged, debilitating illness. In educating ward staff about the unique needs of these patients, we may encourage patience and forbearance as they painstakingly struggle to recover fully. It may also be possible, because of our familiarity with these patients, to help forestall readmission through earlier recognition of re-emergence of old problems.

If resources allowed we could transfer all intensive care patients to high-dependency units to continue their recovery, while still providing a better level of support and care than is available on general wards. But as Bion (1995) remarks there is a serious shortage of facilities for intermediate care because of constraints on resources. If we can support this shortfall through provision of a follow-up service that can improve the quality of care and perhaps prevent the development of further complications for our patients, then we can do no less for them.

Ward visits after intensive care discharge: who could do them?

The consultant on call traditionally did our own follow-up service of patients discharged from intensive care for each day as an extension of the daily ward round. This service was provided in conjunction with the extensive research work being done in the unit, where ward visits by the researchers also often flagged up problems with the patients who might require critical care advice. In addition, the unit has for many years provided a follow-up clinic, seeing patients at 8 weeks and 6 months post-discharge, which provided valuable information on how we could change and improve our care, not only while the patient is in the unit, but in the long term.

It was decided that a suitably qualified nurse could quite adequately concentrate on those few vital days post-discharge when patients are at their most vulnerable and at risk of readmission. This would free up valuable consultant time, although it was made clear that they would be immediately available for consultation should it be required.

Because such senior medical staff had provided the service, it was felt that the nurse should also be a reflection of this to make it credible and more acceptable to the organization. Therefore the post role description demanded seniority and lengthy experience in intensive care, in addition to professional and academic qualifications that would meet the Trust's requirements for advanced nursing practice, as essential qualities. The desired standard was for the post holder to have acquired an MSc in Clinical Nursing or equivalent. The curriculum for this course included the teaching of history-taking and clinical examination skills, communication, in addition to more in-depth theory in the usual sciences – anatomy, physiology, pathophysiology, pharmacology, social sciences, etc. It was felt that these skills were an essential requirement for our follow-up service.

A nurse-led follow-up service does not automatically require this level of qualities and experience. There are organizations where more junior and less qualified members of the intensive care staff are providing a more than adequate service. However, the role boundaries must be clear and unambiguous to protect staff, and the lines of responsibility must be agreed. Junior staff should never be put in the position of having to work beyond their capabilities or responsibility, and as a consequence, the expectations of the service and service providers should be clearly delineated to the satisfaction and agreement of all involved. The level of follow-up service should also reflect the needs of each individual organization, in that what works very well in one may not in another because of their unique differences.

The role of the clinical nurse specialist (CNS) in ward visits should be multifaceted. It must be fluid, dynamic and evolving, able to adjust and grow to reflect and complement changes in the service needs of the organization that it serves. It should not be confined to a rigid job description, but one that gives guidance and allows autonomy for the nurse to be able to use initiative in identifying areas that require improvement and seeking proactively and independently to address them. It is very important then that one is quite clear exactly what qualities are desirable in the person or persons chosen for such a post.

However, based on personal and practical experience, the author's view is that the most useful qualities for any nurse endeavouring to provide this sort of service include excellent communication and diplomacy skills, experience in teaching all levels of staff, flexibility, tenacity, assertiveness and, above all, a very good sense of humour. If one has worked at a senior management position within the intensive care unit, leadership qualities and experience with change management will most certainly have already been acquired, but these are also desirable qualities for anyone involved in the introduction of a new service development.

The development of a new nurse-led service that, in effect, crosses traditional clinical and role boundaries, can be challenging, rewarding, but also frustrating at times. It can be viewed as slightly threatening to those who now have ultimate clinical responsibility for these discharged intensive care patients. There may be resistance to the service from medical and nursing staff, perhaps due to traditional role perceptions or even jealousy and resentment. During the initial introduction period, do not expect to always be greeted graciously or with enthusiasm, no matter how beneficial your visit proves to be. Medical and nursing staff may have feelings of inadequacy at being unable to deal with a patient that they feel they should be able to manage without advice and support. Although they may recognize that the help being proffered is useful and of benefit for the patient, they may also resent having to ask for or take it. The challenge for the CNS is to react positively to such incidents, attempting to build relationships through education, shared knowledge and skills and a non-judgemental manner. You will ultimately achieve what is best for your patients, empowering those who are now providing that care so that the standard is improved for further discharges, but also introducing a culture of openness and sharing of information, where staff will not be afraid actively to seek your help in the future.

Ward visits after intensive care discharge: who should be reviewed?

In our organization all patients discharged from the intensive care unit and those from the high-dependency unit still considered to be at some risk of deterioration, receive a ward visit on the day after discharge. When there are a number of patients to be seen, priority is given to those who have been discharged precipitously, and in particular, those who have been transferred during the night. The main concern is to ensure that no acute deterioration has occurred during the initial period on the ward that may require immediate intervention and/or readmission to the critical care units. The next step is usually to check that the appropriate documentation has accompanied the patient to the ward and that a thorough nursing and medical handover has been done – both verbally and written. Any deficiencies or discrepancies can usually be rectified immediately and documented in the patient's notes or communicated verbally to the receiving medical team. It is also important to check that all of the appropriate members of the multidisciplinary team who need to be involved in the patient's continuing management are aware of the transfer.

Of these, perhaps the chest physiotherapist will be the most important, given the significant number of patients readmitted to intensive care due to respiratory problems. In fact a fairly recent study by Kirby and Durbin (1996) found that the introduction of a respiratory assessment team enabled developing respiratory problems to be identified much earlier in discharged intensive care patients. It was felt that more rapid readmission to intensive care was achieved when it was felt to be necessary, which was also thought to have contributed to decreased mortality rates in these patients. For those of us who do not have the benefit of a dedicated service such as this, the development of a solid relationship with the chest physiotherapy department, building good communication links and fostering a team approach to the management of these patients can only contribute to improving the quality of care patients receive. It helps to ensure that the continuity of the patients' treatment is assured and can be discussed openly on a regular basis to ensure that any deterioration is identified early. The physiotherapist is often the first person thoroughly to assess newly discharged patients to the general ward and acts as a valuable resource in the early identification of new problems, as well as a fresh approach to chronic problems – so long as the bridges have been built and the communication channels are open and based on mutual respect.

The next step is to visit the patient inviting them to voice any concerns or problems they or their family might have now they are back on a general ward. If family members are not with the patient at the time of the CNS's visit, a message is left with the patient or named nurse inviting them to arrange to be seen if there are any issues that they wish to discuss.

Very often you will find that emotions are mixed – anxiety, fear, vulnerability, in addition to relief that a life-threatening event has now passed and a longing to be well enough to go home. Patients who have had a lengthy stay on intensive care can often feel the most lost and abandoned as they may well have become dependent on the closeness and security provided by the intensive care staff. They also find it difficult to understand why they feel so weak and frail, particularly if they remember little of their protracted stay on the unit. It is important to spend time with these patients and attempt to promote more realistic expectations about their continuing recovery, encouraging independence, but always at an achievable pace. It may also help to discuss their stay in the intensive care unit in order to help clarify things and help them to understand why they are so frail, but only if they wish to do so. Some patients are still not ready at this early stage to be reminded of these events or have the lost time filled in for them and this must be respected.

Ward staff may also have mixed feelings about caring for a newly discharged intensive care patient as studies have identified that they find it stressful (Hall-Smith et al., 1997). They are often concerned and apprehensive about receiving such a patient, particularly if they are still relatively nursing dependent by the ward's standards, or have unfamiliar lines or tubes still in place that may require specialist management. Whittaker and Ball (2000) found that the grade of the staff receiving the patient also made a difference to the sort of concerns that were evidenced, with more senior staff more ambivalent towards the patient's immediate problems and more concerned with staffing levels and long-term problems. However, personal experience would suggest that, overall, few ward staff truly welcome a patient transferred from intensive care as they find them too demanding and blame the ICU staff for making the patient dependent on one-to-one care. Patients are also very often frightened by the lack of visibility of the staff and do want the reassurance of knowing that someone is near. This is even more important if they are still so weak as to require full help for activities of daily living and realize that they may have to wait their turn to have these needs met, no matter how urgent they may seem to themselves. It is vitally important to act as the envoy in these situations and try to bring understanding and more realistic expectations on both sides. The patient and his family may gradually be brought to understand that the workload, staffing levels, etc. on the ward cannot support the close monitoring that they had become used to, but also that it really is no longer necessary. The ward staff can be educated to understand the effects of a critical illness, both mentally and physically, on a patient, in order to have greater insight into why they are so slow to recover physical strength and independence. They may come to realize that their dependence is truly not all psychological, but has its roots in true physical weakness.

At each visit, if any signs of early psychological problems are identified (i.e. complaints of nightmares, delusions, flashbacks, etc) the patient is referred to those members of the intensive care team who have come to specialize in these problems. They offer advice and also practical support and intervention with such patients, providing counselling themselves or advising when more formal care is required, i.e. referral to psychiatry/psychology services.

The patient's observation, fluid balance and drug charts, in addition to any recent blood results, are checked for any abnormalities. The patient will be clinically examined if this is indicated and the results of the visit are documented clearly in the patient's medical record and discussed with the named nurse and ward medical staff if there are issues to be addressed. If a patient has any unfamiliar lines or tubes that the staff are unsure of managing, teaching can usually be given immediately or arrangements made to return at a mutually convenient time to go through that care with as many staff as possible. In an area with quite a number of staff who are unfamiliar with certain aspects of care, this may need to be repeated on a number of occasions, as well as trying to be available for practical trouble-shooting whenever it is required, in an attempt to forestall any major problems or complications.

If the patient's condition is giving any cause for concern which the CNS feels would not be appropriate for the ward staff to have to deal with, advice is immediately sought from the intensive care consultant. Usually, if communication has been good and all the support services are in place, the only decision that has to be made is if and when the patient requires further review. This can vary from several hours, to not requiring another visit unless asked to do so by the ward medical staff. It is entirely left to the clinical judgement of the CNS as to when the patient no longer requires intensive care follow-up.

As with much of this discussion, this section can only serve as a template for how a service might be developed and it does not and cannot fully describe the complex, multidimensional interactions that can occur during a ward visit. All developments should reflect not only the unique, specific needs of its parent organization, but also any financial and manpower restrictions that might also need to be taken into consideration. If structured properly the role will develop and grow to reflect demands of, and changes in, service provision.

Ward visits after intensive care discharge: what else can be achieved?

There are many other things that can be achieved during ward visits that do not even necessarily involve the patient that one has gone to review, but may impact on the level or standard of care given to discharged patients, in addition to those who might become our patients in the future. For instance, many patients leave intensive care still cannulated with lines and tubes that some ward areas may have little experience with managing. The education of ward staff in the use and management of these devices can often forestall the need for readmission. For instance, caring for a patient with a tracheostomy can be frightening for nursing staff who have never seen one, let alone been responsible for managing one. The provision of practical support and teaching for staff can be invaluable, particularly if the CNS can be available to help ward staff troubleshoot problems as they arise. Taking ward staff through a problem practically and theoretically at the time it has occurred can empower them, ensuring that they are more able to deal with that problem again should it recur and giving them the confidence to do it for themselves. Building up this relationship of support and education without being judgemental also ensures that staff are not afraid to approach you for advice about other problems or patients they might have. In this way you often become aware of extremely ill ward patients who may subsequently require admission to intensive care and can often speed up the process by speaking to ward medical staff and encouraging them to make a referral. Sometimes all that is required is advice on the patient's medical management or the care of their monitoring lines, etc.

For example, during the initial period of establishing the CNS role in our organization, the major problem referred pertained to central line care and management.

Case study 1

While I was reviewing a discharged surgical patient I was asked by ward staff to look at the central line of a postoperative patient that they were concerned about as it appeared to be blocked. The line had been in for 7 days and it was envisaged that the patient would require it for the foreseeable future as he required intravenous nutrition, antibiotics, blood products, electrolyte supplements and numerous other fluids/drugs. I had assumed from the patient's history and the number of infusions he required that he would have a multilumen cannula sited, but when I investigated, he only had a single lumen cannula that was well and truly blocked.

For those of us who use these lines every day and are also used to patients who require multiple therapy, it would appear to be patently obvious that more than one line was required. We would not only know that most of these infusions should never run concurrently due to incompatibilities, but also from the perspective of introduction of infection. But for inexperienced ward staff, these things are never so clear cut or easily solved. This patient had no other intravenous access. The medical staff who prescribed all these infusions was aware of that fact, but insisted that nursing staff try to administer them all. At the root of the whole problem was the inescapable fact that there were only very junior medical staff available who had no experience of inserting central lines so could not re-site the cannula for a multilumen one. The patient had very poor peripheral access having been in hospital for many weeks and having had numerous cannulations, so that even for products that could be given peripherally, there was no available route.

There were a number of opportunities here for staff and service development. Nursing and medical staff could be educated about the appropriate use of central lines and the fluids that could be given through them. In addition, some thought was given about the most appropriate way to manage such an ill patient, looking at his total needs and how to address them more efficiently. Finally, the issue of unavailability of appropriately trained staff able to insert central lines when required was examined. In this case, the patient would obviously suffer for the lack of foresight regarding his intravenous needs as he now had no access at all and would remain so for an indefinite period of time while suitable personnel were identified who might be able to insert a new line. During all this time he would be unable to have his fluids/drugs and might suffer some consequences as a result. Larger hospitals probably do not have to deal with this sort of problem, employing greater numbers of very experienced staff. We did not even have the benefit of a Nutrition Team who may have been able to assist with the problem of intravenous access. This was obviously not a problem that could be solved immediately or even completely, involving as it did the service provision of a procedure requiring a degree or experience and expertise.

With the support of my consultant mentor, I trained to insert peripherally inserted central catheters (PICC), with the expectation of being able to offer this service to the hospital, not just for our transferred patients but also for patients requiring long-term fluids, nutrition, antibiotics, etc. In this way ward staff had an identifiable person whom they could access to help them with the problem of maintaining central access, especially if it was required for lengthy periods. These products can be left in for much longer than conventional central lines, can also provide more than one lumen for access and have fewer complications during and after insertion. It makes them a fairly safe and reliable product that is user friendly and less likely to cause trepidation on the part of the staff having to manage them. I have encouraged their use earlier in a patient's stay in hospital, if long-term intravenous access is envisaged, to improve the quality of care these patients receive by reducing the number of cannulations they require. Their success in the management of patients requiring long-term parenteral nutrition has also been rapidly proven reducing the need for conventional central line access and the need for experienced personnel to insert them.

This has been a service development that has occurred in response to a need that has been identified within one particular organization. Although we are still left with a need for more personnel experienced in conventional central line insertion, an alternative is now available that may help in many instances of patient management. A CNS doing follow-up work will have the opportunity to identify any number of problem areas, particularly regarding procedures, protocols or standards that may need addressing with a view to change or improvement. Through proactively addressing such issues the standard of care to all patients can be improved, which has implications for those who do not yet require intensive care but who may also be prevented from having to do so.

Over a period of time, the clinical nurse specialist becomes familiar with all the wards in their particular hospital and is able to identify their strengths and weaknesses in care delivery. In doing so specific areas can be targeted for more in-depth teaching that is made available at a time that is convenient for ward staff. This informal approach to education provision can support and enforce more formal, regular and on-going lectures in the classroom made available to all. What has also been useful in our organization has been the ability to offer a rotation for ward staff to work on the high-dependency unit for a 6-week period utilizing a structured practical and theoretical timetable, so that the theory is always supported by guided and supervised practice over a concentrated period. The staff can also return for weekly refreshers a year later. This has been far more beneficial in not only breaking down the barriers between the critical care units and general wards but also in improving the knowledge base of staff by being able to offer concentrated hands-on experience. This does far more for retention of knowledge than the efforts of a single person providing teaching, either in the ward area or in the classroom. Ward staff are able to improve not only their ability to manage complex lines, tubes and monitoring, but also become more aware of how to recognize a patient who is becoming, or has the potential to become, seriously ill. In addition, staff who have rotated to the areas are more willing to ring for advice about patients when the CNS is not available because they are speaking to people with whom they have built up a relationship and who will not feel they are inadequate for seeking help.

Ward visits after intensive care discharge: what does the future hold?

In summary, the clinical nurse specialist can help to promote continuity of care for discharged intensive care patients, ensuring it is seamless and progressive. She can seek to improve communication channels between the critical care areas and general wards, attempting to break down the barriers that have always existed between specialist and general areas. The experience for patients, their families and ward staff can be improved also with good communication and promotion of understanding on both sides. It may be possible to identify patients at risk of deterioration much sooner than would normally have been the case, advising on their management so that they may be safely kept on the ward, or facilitating earlier admission to intensive care should that be required. Areas of potential for improvement can also be identified with the CNS offering advice or practical solutions that will help to facilitate changes in service delivery that positively impact on care delivery. But the cornerstone of any follow-up service provided by nurses will emphasize education, both practical and theoretical, as a means to improve the care of our patients. In providing a highly approachable, effective resource for ward nursing and medical staff seriously ill patients in general wards are also often brought to the CNS's attention for advice on management, although earlier referral to intensive care may be the final decision, on assessment.

It is this final aspect of the role that has become the most recent potential innovation for all hospitals since the publication of the government documents 'Critical to Success' (Audit Commission, 1999) and 'Comprehensive Critical Care' (2000). Similar to other organizations we must also formalize and expand this aspect of our follow-up care to bring us in line with government recommendations on the provision of 'Outreach Care'. The emphasis here is on improving services for patients on wards who are at risk of deteriorating into a need for critical care through a service led by highly experienced critical care personnel, but with the support of an identified multidisciplinary team. It is envisaged that devolving critical care skills and knowledge to ward staff will enhance their ability to identify and manage critically ill patients, facilitating earlier admission to intensive care or averting admission altogether. In most instances scoring systems (i.e. Early Warning Score; Morgan *et al.*, 1997), based on changes in clinical signs as a predictor of clinical deterioration, are being introduced as one method of assisting staff in the identification of ill patients. Once a patient has been identified, ward staff can call on the outreach team to advise them on the care of that patient. The education and sharing of critical care skills is essential so that ward staff become more proficient at managing these patients themselves, improving the service to intensive care discharges as well as those identified as potential patients for critical care. The follow-up of discharged intensive care patients is still highlighted as a priority so that the continuing recovery of these patients is assured.

Our hospital has been at the forefront of developments and improvements in the care and service provision for critically ill patients, mostly due to the efforts of Drs Griffiths and Jones. They have pioneered the concept of follow-up care for these patients that has been greeted with scepticism by some, but with very real enthusiasm and support by those who really care about these patients and the quality of the service that we provide for them.

It is through research such as theirs (e.g. Jones, 2001) that the need for a structured physical rehabilitation programme for patients has proven to be yet another valuable tool in improving recovery from intensive care. In conjunction with, and under the supervision of the researcher it is envisaged that it may be part of the role of our Outreach Team to administer and monitor the effectiveness of these rehabilitation programmes for all suitable intensive care patients – something that has been impossible for only one person to achieve given the escalating number of patients requiring our services each year. It is hoped that in allowing nearly all our intensive care patients and their families to participate in this structured programme, it will enhance their recovery from a critical illness and also improve our ability to ensure that these patients stand the best chance of a continuing positive trajectory on the recovery continuum and reduce their chances of requiring readmission. It may also act as an important adjunct to the education needs of ward staff in achieving an understanding and insight into the special requirements of intensive care patients and their families.

For those who are truly passionate about critical care, the commitment to improving the experience for patients and their families will most certainly not stop here. Through research, audit and comparison of our results nationally and internationally, we will continue to strive to achieve the best service for our patients. The role of the clinical nurse specialist in the provision of ward follow-up is a small, yet extremely valuable addition to the armoury that we have to help deal with the problems faced by patients recovering from critical illness, in addition to those who have yet to require our services. It is a role that should never be viewed in isolation as its very strengths lie in the ability to identify and liaise with the most appropriate members of the multidisciplinary team in order to achieve a seamless, quality standard of care for patients.

The future can only continue to bring further exciting and challenging opportunities for all of us committed to caring for and improving our care for critically ill patients.

References

Audit Commission (1999) *Critical to Success. The place of efficient and effective critical care services within the acute hospital.* Audit Commission, London: October 1999.

Baigelman W, Katz R, Geary G Patient readmission to critical care units during the same hospitalization at a community teaching hospital. *Intensive Care Medicine* 1983; **9**, 253–6.

Biley FC Effects of noise in hospitals. *British Journal of Nursing* 1994; **3**, 110–12.

Bion J Rationing intensive care. *British Medical Journal* 1995; **310**, 682–3.

Bone RC, McElwee NE, Eubanks DH, Gluck EH Analysis of indications for early discharge from the intensive care unit. *Chest* 1993; **104**(6), 1813–17.

Chen LM, Martin CM, Keenan SP *et al.* Patients readmitted to the intensive care unit during the same hospitalisation: clinical features and outcomes. *Critical Care Medicine* 1998; **26**(11), 1834–41.

Comprehensive Critical Care (2000) *Report of an Expert Group.* Department of Health, London.

Compton P Critical illness and intensive care: what it means to the client. *Critical Care Nurse* 1991; **11**, 50–6.

Cutler L, Garnet M Reducing relocation stress after discharge from the intensive therapy unit. *Intensive and Critical Care Nursing* 1995; **11**, 333–5.

Durbin CG, Kopel RF A case-control study of patients readmitted to the intensive care unit. *Critical Care Medicine* 1993; **21**(10), 1547–53.

Franklin C, Jackson D Discharge decision-making in a medical ICU: Characteristics of unexpected readmissions. *Critical Care Medicine* 1983; **11**(2), 61–6.

Goldfrad C, Rowan K Consequences of discharges from intensive care at night. *Lancet* 2000; **355**, 1138–42.

Goldhill DR, Sumner A Outcome of intensive care patients in a group of British intensive care units. *Critical Care Medicine* 1998; **26**(8), 1337–45.

Griffiths RD, Jones C, Macmillan RR Where is the harm in not knowing? Care after intensive care. *Clinical Intensive Care* 1996; **7**, 144–5.

Hall-Smith J, Ball C, Coakley J Follow-up services and the development of a clinical nurse specialist in intensive care. *Intensive and Critical Care Nursing* 1997; **13**, 243–8.

Jones C Rehabilitation following critical illness, support for patients. *Unpublished PhD Thesis*, University of Liverpool, 2001.

Jones C, Griffiths RD Identifying post intensive care patients who may need physical rehabilitation. *Clinical Intensive Care* 2000; **11**(1), 35–8.

Jones C, Humphris GM, Griffiths RD Psychological morbidity following critical illness – the rationale for care after intensive care. *Clinical Intensive Care* 1998; **9**, 199–205.

Kirby EG, Durbin CG Establishment of a respiratory assessment team is associated with decreased mortality in patients re-admitted to the ICU. *Respiratory Care* 1996; **41**(10), 903–7.

Lloyd G Psychological problems and the intensive care unit. *British Medical Journal* 1993; **307**, 458–9.

Mata GV, Fernandez RR, Aragon AP *et al*. Analysis of quality of life in polytraumatized patients two years after discharge from an intensive care unit. *Journal of Trauma* 1996; **41**(2), 326–32.

Morgan RJM, Williams F, Wright MM An early warning scoring system for detecting developing critical illness. *Clinical Intensive Care* 1997; **8**, 100.

Ridley SA Intermediate care. *Anaesthesia* 1998; **52**, 654–64.

Rubins HB, Moskowitz MA Discharge decision making in a medical intensive care unit. *American Journal of Medicine* 1988; **84**, 863–9.

Saarmann L Transfer out of critical care: freedom or fear? *Critical Care Nurse Quarterly* 1993; **16**(1), 78–85.

Smith S, Garnett P, Buckley P Delirium in the critically ill. *Care of the Critically Ill* 1997; **13**, 175–8.

Wallis CB, Davies HTO, Shearer AJ Why do patients die on general wards after discharge from intensive care units? *Anaesthesia* 1997; **52**, 9–14.

Whittaker J, Ball C Discharge from intensive care: a view from the ward. *Intensive and Critical Care Nursing* 2000; **16**, 135–43.

The ICU team on the ward after discharge: case studies

John Coakley, Shelagh Platt and Jess Townsend

Introduction

For many patients, admission to an ICU constitutes only a brief interlude in their period of care, and it would be inappropriate for the ICU team to have any significant input into their care after they have returned to the ward. Nevertheless, there are some patients who, for reasons of disease severity or duration of stay, do warrant continuing review from the ICU team.

Problems were outlined to us by several patients during the early weeks of our ICU follow-up clinic which made us think that ward follow-up would have been helpful. As a Senior Registrar in Respiratory Medicine, one of the authors saw patients with a variety of respiratory conditions who had spent variable amounts of time on ICUs. These patients often had questions for which it was clear that the non-ICU-trained doctor would have difficulty providing answers.

The changing nature of medical and nursing training, and alterations in the provision of patient care have also resulted in potential difficulty. In the UK, medical training has become much more focused on developing a speciality, and there is concern in some quarters that the care of the patients with problems of a generalist nature is being neglected. The provision of nursing care is also developing a more specialist focus, and many experienced nurses are now developing skills as clinical nurse specialists and nurse consultants, or perhaps moving into management and administrative posts. The loss of this experienced tier of nursing talent from the general wards may cause problems. There has also been an increasing proportion of sicker patients on the wards compared with the situation 10 or 20 years ago. There has not generally been a commensurate increase in nursing staff levels or skill-mix.

It is also worth remembering that the financial, medical, nursing and sometimes emotional investment that has gone into supporting a patient who has progressed from being critically ill to being in a state of readiness for the wards has been substantial. It is sometimes difficult to relinquish the care of these patients, and it is often difficult for the patients and their relatives to adjust to a new set of doctors and nurses.

For the reasons outlined above it may be appropriate for ICU staff to follow-up a selected population of patients discharged from the ICU in order to provide continuity of care. The rest of this chapter describes some scenarios from the authors' experience in which intervention from ICU staff has been helpful and some where lack of involvement of ICU staff has led to problems.

Case study 1

A 45-year-old male was transferred from another hospital having undergone a colectomy for carcinoma of the colon. He had developed septic shock following an anastomotic breakdown, for which he underwent laparotomy with formation of a colostomy. His course on the ICU had been stormy, and during the course of his stay he had been enrolled in a study of a novel agent designed to reverse hypotension in septic shock. Part of the requirement of this study was that the patients were followed-up, and one of our research fellows visited him at home. During the course of the visit it became apparent that he had a number of questions, complaints and psychological difficulties. He had not been offered an appointment at our ICU outpatient clinic because he lived a long distance from the hospital, and was anyway already under the care of the hospital from which he had been referred originally. In the light of our research fellow's observations, the patient was offered a clinic appointment, which he accepted. A number of difficulties were outlined, which it might be helpful to consider under different headings. These findings have led us to change a number of our policies surrounding ICU discharge and ward follow-up.

The most disturbing aspect of the patient's perception of his ICU stay was his conviction that he had been abducted by the Spanish authorities, and was being pumped full of illegal drugs. Furthermore, he was being used in anti-drug propaganda films while being held prisoner in a train tunnel. He also remembered that a nurse had performed an unauthorized operation upon him.

These feelings had caused him considerable distress for some weeks, although at the time of review he was gradually coming to terms with them.

These seemingly bizarre delusions all had rational explanations, given that the patient had no memory of the second operation or of the transfer to another hospital. As he emerged from sedation he had to try to come to some understanding of what had happened to him. At the time of his ICU stay there were two Spanish doctors working on the unit, and they not unnaturally spoke Spanish from time to time. The patient thus imagined that he was in Spain.

It is common for patients to receive analgesia as a narcotic infusion, and we use morphine for most patients. This is usually administered using a syringe driver with a 60 ml syringe. As the patient became vaguely aware of his surroundings, he noticed that the people around him were passing round enormous syringes saying 'here's the morphine for Mr X'.

During his stay with us, there was a crisis of ICU bed provision, and a news programme came to interview the director of the ICU on the unit. Although the patient himself was not filmed, and was apparently sedated he had clearly been aware of the presence of the TV cameras and constructed his own explanation.

He had known he was trapped in a train tunnel because he was in darkness, and could see flashing red and green lights, with occasional bursts of white light. ICUs are noisy places, and one of our noise reduction measures has been to turn off the ringing tones on the ICU telephones. The three telephone extensions for the unit have coded flashing lights; red, green and white. Most people use the red and green numbers.

This patient was aware of his first operation, an elective procedure for which he had signed a consent form, and remembered recovering from surgery without a colostomy. Imagine his surprise to discover that a member of the nursing staff (who was in fact changing the colostomy bag) was interfering in his lower abdomen, apparently fashioning a colostomy for which he had not given his consent.

These experiences had not been described by the patient at all during his lengthy post-ICU hospital stay, indeed, on review on the ward he had seemed rather withdrawn. It is perhaps not surprising that the patient was not prepared to talk about his experiences to the people who had been responsible for keeping him in these rather strange surroundings. He was not even sure whether his wife had been part of the plot or not, since he had been aware of her presence during this enforced captivity. We have modified our approach to patients on the ward after discharge from ICU since this episode, and an example of this is given later.

The patient's psychological troubles were worrying enough, but there were also physical problems arising as a result of his catabolic illness, which caused considerable problems on the ward. The first was the severe weakness, which had delayed his weaning from ventilatory support. Once he was able to breathe unaided, his endotracheal tube was removed and he was discharged to the ward the next day. He seemed to be making good progress on ward follow-up, but when he attended the clinic he told us that it was common on the ward for his meals to be brought to him and left in front of him with a knife and fork. When the domestic staff came to clear up, they usually commented 'not hungry today then', and removed his plate. He was physically incapable of lifting cutlery, and could not feed himself. This incapacity had not been made clear to staff on the ward.

The other major concern that the patient had was that no-one explained to him that his physical appearance had altered during the course of his stay on the ICU. He was thus greatly disturbed to be confronted with his new facial features when a well-intentioned member of staff on the ward showed him into the bathroom so that he could shave in front of a mirror.

These diverse problems which faced the patient both in the immediate aftermath of his ICU stay and also following his discharge home caused considerable distress to him and his wife. By the time he came to see us in the clinic 6 months later, these problems were starting to resolve themselves, but he clearly felt the need to come and talk to us about them. It is our belief that had we employed a more proactive approach to this problem, some of them might have been avoided. It was clear that no-one from his referring team had offered any explanation to him, and indeed it is unlikely that anyone asked.

Case study 2

A 39-year-old female was admitted following a laparotomy for peritonitis. She developed raised intra-abdominal pressure with respiratory, cardiovascular and renal failure. Repeat laparotomy was necessary and she returned to the unit with an open abdomen, but otherwise improving. She then developed sepsis and disseminated intravascular coagulation with severe thrombocythaemia. As this recovered, there was rebound thrombocythaemia. At around this time gross facial and upper limb swelling became obvious, and a clinical diagnosis of superior vena caval obstruction was made which was subsequently confirmed radiologically. Heparin therapy was instituted, but satisfactory anticoagulation was difficult to achieve. After 2 weeks, the facial swelling subsided sufficiently for her trachea to be extubated.

She was discharged to a general ward. As part of her follow-up by the ICU team, she was specifically asked about peculiar dreams or experiences she might wish to talk about. She was able to discuss several of these, including a feeling of abduction and imprisonment and a clear recollection of men and women gathering at the end of her bed to talk about how to kill her. After a few days, the distress she suffered from these experiences had diminished, and she no longer found them threatening. She also needed support and reassurance that her physical progress, agonizingly slow as she perceived it, was in fact normal.

At this time (being an extended public holiday) she was seen by a different member of the referring discipline every day, and felt a lack of confidence in them. None of them knew her or her family. For several days, the only continuity in her care was provided by the ICU team, who were also the only people who could obtain blood samples to check her anticoagulation because of difficult venous access.

Case study 3

An elderly man with a history of chronic lung disease and presumed excessive alcohol intake fell down the stairs at home. He presented the next day to the A&E Department, and was initially admitted to a general ward having sustained several right-sided rib fractures. Over the next 24 h he developed progressive respiratory distress and was referred to the ICU team. In view of his rapidly deteriorating respiratory function, mechanical ventilation was instituted. Despite this he developed increasing hypoxaemia and elevated peak airway pressures. Chest radiographs showed unilateral injury, and he was therefore treated with differential lung ventilation. This proved successful, and he was eventually weaned onto conventional mechanical ventilation, facilitated by a tracheostomy. He spent a total of 50 days on the ICU before he could breathe satisfactorily, but was eventually discharged to a general medical ward. He had been assessed by the speech and language therapists because of difficulty in swallowing. They had suggested that he be kept nil-by-mouth with his tracheostomy cuff inflated and nutrition maintained with nasoenteric feed. He was also being followed-up on the ward by the physiotherapists for both locomotor and respiratory assistance. Sadly, he had become rather depressed, and feared that he would never leave hospital. He persuaded the nursing and medical staff on the ward that since he was going to die anyway, he might as well die eating and drinking normally. He was allowed generous access to liquids. The ICU registrar was summoned urgently one breakfast time, when the patient's oxygen saturation had fallen to 70%. The appropriate action was taken and the instructions about tracheostomy care were reinforced.

Summary

One of the major alterations we have made to discharge planning from the ICU to the ward is based on the observation that ICU nurses and ward staff used the same words to mean very different things. For instance, the phrase 'this patient has done really well' means to the ICU staff 'is lucky to be alive, and can now just breathe unaided'. To ward staff, it means 'is nearly ready for home'. This enormous difference in meaning has significant implications for the way the patient is treated. The handover is now structured to emphasize that 'this patient has just survived a major life-threatening illness, and is the sickest patient you will have on the ward'. This has produced a major alteration in the way these patients are perceived by ward staff, and made them feel more comfortable about contacting the ICU team.

The efficacy in terms of outcomes is harder to quantify. Much of the support that can be given is psychological, and it is always difficult to measure this. There is no doubt that patients, their relatives and ward staff feel better about having some sort of continuity provided by the regular visits from the ICU team. Whether such an approach can improve physical outcomes is more uncertain. There is no doubt in our minds that the supervision of devices common in the ICU (tracheostomy tubes, mini-tracheostomies, central lines, parenteral nutrition and so on) is helpful to staff on general wards where experience of and exposure to such devices is limited.

Furthermore, it has been shown that doctors outside the ICU sometimes fail to appreciate the life-threatening nature of physical signs and symptoms. These failings usually relate to a lack of awareness of the predictors of sudden death, such as failure to protect the airway, impending respiratory failure or circulatory embarrassment (McGloin et al., 1997; McQuillan et al., 1998). If such failures can occur before admission to ICU, then they are presumably likely to occur afterwards. The death rate among patients discharged from the ICU is such that there can be no cause for complacency about providing satisfactory follow-up arrangements. If this means that the ICU doctors and nurses have to get out and about in the hospital, so be it. They might even be able to spot the deteriorating patient, who has not yet visited the ICU but needs to, a little bit earlier.

References

McGloin H, Adam S, Singer M The quality of pre-ICU care influences outcome of patients admitted from the ward. *Clinical Intensive Care* 1997; **8**, 104.

McQuillan P, Pilkington S, Allan A *et al*. Confidential inquiry into quality of care before admission to intensive care. *British Medical Journal* 1998; **316**, 1853–8.

Setting up a doctor-led clinic

Carl Waldmann

Introduction

Whether an ICU follow-up should be doctor- or nurse-led is a matter for discussion. We are seeing the boundaries of responsibility between doctor and nurse in specialist areas becoming less distinct. There is no reason why such a clinic cannot be run by a critical nurse specialist or one of the new breed of nurse consultants. So far as our clinic in Reading is concerned, we conduct a clinic run jointly by a sister and doctor (Figure 9.1) with a passion for the follow-up programme.

The sister recruits the patients, the doctor conducts the interviews at the clinic and the sister then organizes the return of questionnaires, counselling and visits to the ICU and also will write diaries for the patients. Recently, the sister's role has developed and includes undertaking home visits.

Initially the clinic took place in an informal room close to the ICU, but as it grew it was eventually accommodated in the outpatient department. The advantage of this is that we could use outpatient's infrastructure for booking appointments and retrieving notes.

In a recent Linkman survey on follow-up there were 61 replies, 10 hospitals said they have a clinic up and running, 10 were about to start one and 41 had no plans. Of the 10 with a clinic, five were nurse-led and four doctor-led or really nurse and doctor-led. In one hospital a researcher conducted follow-up by telephone. The overall number of patients seen were from 2 to 20 per month.

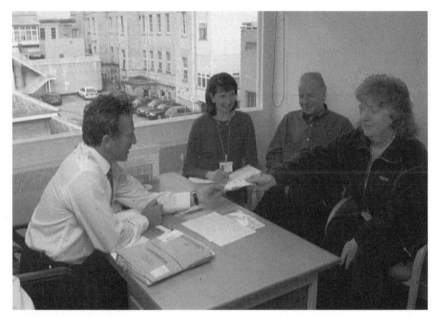

Figure 9.1 Clinic visit

Getting started

1 Identifying clerical and IT support

At the moment our information is entered onto a specially designed questionnaire, rather than in the patient's notes. After three visits (one year) a discharge summary is written and entered into the formal notes. With the acquisition of a clinical information system in our ICU, the intention is to add follow-up details directly onto the ICU patient's file, so that it is available to any clinician in ICU, should he or she wish to know the progress of a patient. Ideally, in the future, when the hospital is networked, we hope to be able to plug a laptop computer into any outpatient room and directly enter a patient's details of progress into a database, making analysis easy. Clerical support is required for writing referral letters to other specialists and progress letters to the GPs.

2 Support from GPs and hospital colleagues

It is imperative to inform other hospital specialists, as well as patients' GPs, that this service is available in addition to the service they already provide. There is nothing more annoying than arranging an outpatient appointment for an ex-ICU patient who may have seen his surgeon one day previously, or referring a patient for further treatment without the knowledge of the GP.

3 Arrange transport if necessary

The hospital transport is available for outpatient appointments, but is rarely requested. To our surprise, patients who found themselves in our ICU out of their area (out of area transfer (OATS)) are keen enough to attend follow-up from as far as Southend and Milton Keynes.

4 Arrange for appropriate investigations

The investigations we employ more regularly are:

● swabs for MRSA
● pulmonary function tests
● creatinine clearance
● MRI trachea post-tracheostomy (Figure 9.2)

5 Counselling

Our ICU follow-up sister is responsible for counselling the patients with post-traumatic stress disorder. However, if it is apparent that further help is required,

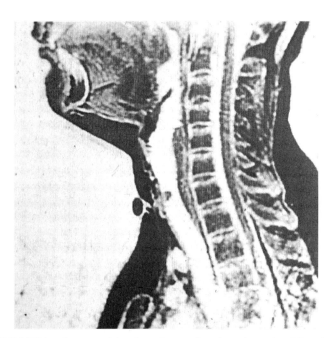

Figure 9.2 MRI trachea post-tracheostomy showing stenosis at level of tracheostomy

we are able to request the services of a liaison psychiatrist without attaching too much stigma to such a referral.

6 Rehabilitation

In a recent study it has been demonstrated that, using a self-directed graded exercise programme, physical recovery from critical illness can be significantly hastened (Jones *et al.*, 2001).

There are already rehabilitation programmes for patients with cardiac, respiratory and neurological problems. We intend to extend these rehabilitation services to patients who have endured a stay in the intensive care unit. In spite of the fact that many have had multisystem failure, there is no specific programme for such patients.

Referring patients to other services

Many patients seen in our clinic do need further specialist care. They often feel more comfortable discussing their problems at our clinic rather than with their GP and usually find it easier to be referred on. This may present a dilemma, in that if it is considered necessary to refer on, it needs to be done with the full knowledge and permission of the patient's GP. We have rarely seen any conflict in this area.

In a sample of 44 patients, who survived ICU with multisystem dysfunction, a total of 26 referrals were made (Wilkins *et al.*, 1998).

The main specialities to which patients are referred are:

1 ENT

A small percentage of patients require revision of their percutaneous tracheostomy scar, this can easily be done in the ENT outpatient department under local anaesthesia. One of the difficulties we had was a conflict with the District Priorities Group, who decided that as this was a cosmetic procedure, they would not fund it. This decision was eventually reversed.

2 Pain clinic

Patients who have had a protracted stay in ICU and have developed critical care myopathy and neuropathy, may develop severe pain in their joints. One such patient requiring ICU for 6 months due to pancreatitis, responded to guanethidine Bier's Block for pain around his ankle.

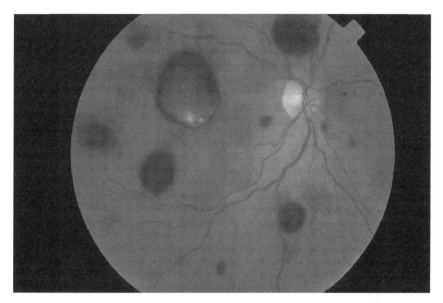

Figure 9.3 Retinal damage requiring referral for laser therapy

3 Ophthalmology

Of particular interest was one patient who had reduced visual activity following a cardiac arrest. This responded to laser therapy and the patient was able to drive again (Figure 9.3).

4 Dermatology

A group of our patients developed intractable pruritus, lasting 6 months post-intensive care. Eventually it was ascertained that the regular use of starch during their ICU stay may have been a contributing factor.

5 Neurology

We have referred patients who, in the year post-ICU, have developed parkinsonism.

6 Rehabilitation physician

The Department of Rehabilitation Medicine has been particularly useful for patients with cognitive deficit following head injury and meningitis. These patients receive help with memory dysfunction and relatives are advised that too early a resumption of a university degree may be inappropriate.

7 Andrology clinic

Significant numbers of male patients suffer impotence and have benefitted from referral to psychosexual counselling and urologists (see Chapter 4 on Sexual Dysfunction).

8 Other

We have also been able to refer patients for extra help from social services, physiotherapy and health visitors. We have often found that some of our patients are caught in a bureaucratic trap and are unable to get out of it because of apathy and weakness to chase what they are rightfully entitled to. Making one or two phone calls to various social services on behalf of the patient may well ruffle a few feathers.

Benefits to patients

In order to ascertain whether our clinic was useful to patients we conducted a survey among all patients discharged from the follow-up clinic one year after ICU discharge (Hames *et al.*, 2001). There was a 99% response rate to the questionnaire (65/66). All but one patient admitted they had benefitted from the follow-up programme:

- 80% could have questions answered
- 76% could discuss their problems
- 94% would recommend the follow-up to friends
- 26% benefitted from counselling
- 28% benefitted from referral to other specialists
- 48% felt they were helping ICU staff
- 24% appreciated receiving a diary of events while on ICU.

Most patients commented on the lack of step-down facility on leaving ICU and going to the ward and several commented on their concern at being unable to communicate with staff on ICU, the majority of whom were unable to lip read.

Benefits to staff

All the ICU staff have been delighted with the feedback they have received from the clinic and all members attend at least one clinic. The ways in which ward rounds are conducted, care about dignity of the patients and any concerns that they may be aware of, have all been highlighted. We have been able to increase the number of windows in the ICU and are putting up clocks at the end of the beds.

Most patients are grateful and have made generous donations specifically for ICU. One such donation from a grateful patient's employer paid for a blood gas machine.

Cost

The costs are set out in Table 9.1.

Table 9.1 Costs

Nursing	G Grade salary for 37.5 hours per week • time to visit patients on the ward and at home • two or more clinics per month • counselling • teaching and feeding back information to other staff	£18 000
Medical	One consultant session per week	£6 000
Administration	10 hours per week • appointments • coordinating clinic appointments • gathering hospital notes	£4 000
Laboratory tests and X-rays	• MRSA swabs • MRI scanning • Blood tests • PFT	£2 000
	Total	**£30 000**

References

Hames KC, Gager M, Waldmann CS Patient satisfaction with specialist ICU Follow-Up. *British Journal of Anaesthesia* 2001; **87**, 372.

Jones C, Skirrow P, Griffiths RD *et al*. Rehabilitation after critical illness: a randomised, controlled trial. *British Journal of Anaesthesia* 2001; **87**(2), 330.

Wilkins A, Koshy G, Waldmann CS Long-term outcome of patients in ICU with multi-organ failure. *British Journal of Anaesthesia* 1998; **81**, 651.

Setting up a nurse-led clinic

Clare Sharland

Introduction

Intensive care patients and relatives, following their discharge from hospital, suffer with significant physical and psychological problems (Jones *et al.*, 1998) that impact on their quality of life. A follow-up service plays an essential role in improving the speed and quality of recovery from critical illness (Audit Commission, 1999; Department of Health, 2000).

Our clinic is multifunctional, providing an invaluable service for former patients and relatives, and improving the quality of care for the future. The service comprises a nurse-led outpatient clinic and individual patient consultations on the ward following intensive care unit (ICU) discharge.

The nurse-led outpatient clinic is held twice a month, but if patients are not able to travel to hospital the follow-up sister visits them at home. The clinic provides support, advice and information for patients and relatives during a stressful time in their lives. Any problems are identified, help offered and appropriate referrals made for specialist advice. Feedback from patients and relatives has initiated changes in clinical practice to improve the quality of care. The ward visits enable the follow-up sister to assess the patient's progress, promote continuity of care, and help identify any long-term problems.

This chapter will discuss the setting up of our outpatient follow-up clinic, including the different components of the service. The benefits of the service for patients and relatives will be apparent throughout the chapter. Finally, evaluation and audit of the service, ward visits and future developments will be discussed.

Background

Our ICU follow-up clinic was set up in 1995, for general intensive care patients from Southampton University Hospitals NHS Trust. The funding for this service originally came from the clinical trial budget, but is now provided from ICU funds. Initially, we wanted to know the answer to some basic questions. What happened to patients after they left intensive care? How long did it take them to recover? What problems did they encounter during their recovery from critical illness? After the clinic had been established for a couple of months, we quickly realized it was not as simple and straightforward as we had first thought. The physical, psychological and social problems experienced by former patients and their relatives were common, complex and varied in severity. Many required further referral and professional intervention.

Getting started

Once the unit had agreed to fund the follow-up service, the first priorities were to identify the staff to run the clinic, the resources required, the patients to attend the clinic, when to invite patients (in respect of timing after their discharge home), how often to run the clinics and where.

Who will run the clinic?

On our unit, we decided a nurse was the most appropriate person to lead the clinic, for many reasons as shown in Table 10.1.

Cost is an important consideration in today's healthcare climate. Nursing time costs less than medical time and therefore had an important part to play in the setting up of the follow-up service.

Cost was not the only factor for a nurse leading our clinic. The knowledge base and clinical expertise of an experienced ICU nurse provided an excellent foundation for this role. Patients and relatives need detailed information about

Table 10.1 Why nurse-led?

- Cost
- Qualifications of the ICU nurse; knowledge base and clinical expertise
- Qualities of a nurse; good communication and interpersonal skills
- Supportive intensive care and hospital consultants

---

their critical illness. An experienced nurse can explain and answer questions, using language that the patient and relative can understand. Clear, non-technical language suitable to the person's age, education and cultural background can facilitate the discussion (Myerscough, 1992).

Good communication and interpersonal skills are an essential quality for an effective interview. A part of this interview involves giving advice and information, but for a significant amount of time the emphasis is on listening. The patient and relative's experiences need to be explored, in order to identify and focus on their problems. Empathy, genuineness and understanding will encourage the person to talk about these areas (Tschudin, 1995). It can be an advantage for the follow-up sister to attain a counselling qualification to support this role. Some people feel more comfortable talking to nursing staff and may feel anxious seeing a doctor. This can prevent them asking questions and influences the retention of information. People forget a third of information given at an outpatient appointment (Ley and Spelman, 1965). It is therefore necessary to make people feel at ease, to repeat information and to ask for feedback to check their understanding of what has been said.

In our experience, people are aware of how pressurized medical time is and therefore do not want to trouble the doctor with a little problem. For example, Mr A, a 60-year-old man, was in ICU for 10 days with pneumonia. While in ICU, he had localized compartment syndrome following a right brachial artery puncture, requiring a fasciotomy and multiple explorations of this arm. Mr A, at his ICU follow-up appointment, explained his main problem was numbness in his right hand. He could not write or drive his car, and suffered with insomnia due to pain in this hand. Mr A had seen his physician at his outpatient appointment, but had no time to discuss it and 'did not want to trouble the busy doctor'. Mr A was re-referred to the orthopaedic surgeon by the ICU follow-up sister and is undergoing investigations for this problem.

Our nurse-led clinic could not function without the support from the intensive care consultants and the other hospital consultants. The ICU consultants are available for advice at any time during or after the clinic. Patients see their own hospital consultant at their routine outpatient appointment for assessment of their medical condition and treatment. If an aspect of their treatment or condition has been overlooked, the hospital consultants have welcomed referrals and feedback from our clinic.

Resources for a follow-up clinic

The resources required for a follow-up service will vary between units, depending on the available budget and the size of the intensive care unit. The resources for our follow-up service are listed in Table 10. 2. We have a seven-bedded general ICU and there are approximately 450 ICU survivors per annum, of whom 80 were in ICU for more than 4 days.

Table 10.2 Resources for a follow-up service

- Experienced ICU nurse
- A room to hold consultation
- Secretarial support
- Computer and photocopier
- Information technology training
- Answer machine for telephone helpline

The running cost of our follow-up service is calculated according to our staff costs. These consist of a G grade sister for 10 hours per week and secretarial support for 5 hours per month.

Our follow-up sister dedicates 10 hours per week to the service. The primary responsibilities of this role include organizing and running one or two follow-up clinics per month, ward visits to patients discharged from ICU, responding to a telephone helpline, writing referral letters, interview synopsis and audit, and feedback and education for unit staff.

The secretarial support is minimal at the present time, due to financial constraints. The secretary has responsibilities for writing letters to patients, their general practitioners and hospital consultants, and for retrieving and returning patients' hospital notes.

Who attends the clinic?

The patient and relative groups attending our follow-up clinic are summarized in Table 10.3. We routinely invite patients who have been on ICU for more than 4 days, together with their relative or close friend. This gives us a manageable number of patients to see each month, within available resources.

ICU or ward staff can refer any patient or relative, irrespective of their length of ICU stay. Any patient or relative can refer themselves by letter or phone and they are informed of the follow-up service in the ICU discharge information. A contact telephone number is clearly written and an answer machine is available.

Table 10.3 Patients attending the clinic

- Patient or relative on ICU more than 4 days
- Patient or relative referred by ICU staff
- Patient or relative referred by ward staff
- Patient or relative self-referral

A relative or close friend is encouraged to attend the clinic appointment for a variety of reasons. Relatives can have psychological and social problems as a result of their traumatic experience. These problems need addressing and some may require referral for professional advice. Relatives contribute to the discussion about the patient's ICU stay and they give valuable feedback about the care received. They may have unanswered questions, which have been worrying them. During the discussions, it is beneficial for the patient and relative to hear the same information together to avoid confusion, reduce the risk of misunderstandings and increase the retention of information.

When to invite patients?

At our clinic, we see patients at 2, 6 and 12 months after intensive care discharge. We invite patients at 2 months after ICU discharge, as this can be the most psychologically stressful phase of critical illness. Patients have had time to reflect on what has happened, they learn how severe their illness has been and how close to death they came (Compton, 1991). They are aware of their physical limitations, and how their behaviour and feelings impact on their family and friends. Relatives can also find the initial stage of recovery very difficult. It is therefore important to hold an outpatient appointment at this time, to identify problems and reduce the risk of a problem deteriorating further. In the case of severe psychological problems, clinical experience suggests that early intervention improves prognosis and, for some cases, prompt recognition of extreme stress can facilitate prevention of post-traumatic stress disorder (PTSD) (Ramsey, 1990).

If a patient is in hospital at 2 months post-ICU discharge, we invite them to attend their first follow-up interview 1 month after their discharge home. This allows time for the patient and their relatives to establish a realistic impression of life at home.

Preparation for the clinic

The preparation for a clinic involves the components stated in Table 10.4. Secretarial support is extremely beneficial at this stage, essentially for writing letters and retrieving medical notes.

Booking a room

The venue for the follow-up clinic is important and may affect the quality of the service provided. A place that is easy for patients to locate is necessary, as they and their relatives may feel anxious about returning to the hospital again. The room environment must be conducive to a relaxed and informal discussion. Communication can be hindered or encouraged by the physical setting. Ideally, the room needs to be warm with good ventilation; quiet with no outside distractions or

Table 10.4 Preparation for the clinic

- Booking a room
- Letter to patient
- Letter to GP and hospital consultant
- Call for medical notes
- Summary of main ICU events
- Designate unit staff member to attend

---

interruptions; private to protect confidentiality; and have no tables or barriers to communication.

Presently, we hold our clinic in a room near the ICU. This has the advantage of conveniently being able to show patients and relatives around the unit. Everyone who has re-visited the unit has found the experience extremely beneficial (visiting the unit is discussed later in the chapter).

Planning clinic list

The organization of the list of clinic patients influences the effectiveness of the clinic. At the first (2 months post-ICU discharge) interview, we allow 1 h for each patient. This ensures patients have time to discuss all parts of the follow-up interview, including visiting the unit. Half an hour is allocated for 6 and 12 month post-ICU discharge interviews. The length of interview will be adjusted if the patient or relative had many problems at their first consultation.

We carefully plan appointments to ensure they do not coincide with other hospital appointments within the same week. This is primarily for the patient's convenience and secondly, because it can otherwise be difficult to retrieve their medical notes.

Appointment letters are sent to the patient 2–3 weeks prior to their appointment and acceptance of the appointment is by letter or telephone. The content of the letter clearly states the aims of the clinic and relatives or friends are encouraged to attend.

We send an informative letter to the patient's general practitioner (GP) and hospital consultant; it states the aims of the clinic, highlights that we will not change treatment initiated by them, and that we will feedback appropriate information.

Retrieving medical notes and summary of main ICU events

Medical notes are retrieved a week prior to the clinic appointment by our secretary. Before the clinic appointment, the ICU follow-up sister writes a summary of the main ICU events. This saves time during the consultation as it can be difficult to locate the important parts of their intensive care stay.

Designate unit staff member to attend

We encourage a member of the unit team to attend the clinic whenever possible. The staff can gain feedback about a patient's health, their feelings and experiences of ICU. Information about a patient's progress can encourage unit staff morale, motivation and job satisfaction (Hackman and Lawler, 1971). Awareness of the patient's perspective is beneficial. It enlightens staff and changes their understanding of patients' and relatives' feelings, which can lead to improvements in clinical practice.

The clinic consultation

The first consultation consists of a comprehensive discussion with the patient and their relative (if present). It aims to incorporate many aspects of their experiences of intensive care and recovery from critical illness, as listed in Table 10.5.

The 6 and 12 month post-ICU discharge interviews concentrate on the health and progress of the patient and their relative. This will include reviewing previous problems and when appropriate, identifying and assessing new problems.

The interviews are very relaxed and informal. Note taking during the interview is kept to a minimum, as it inhibits communication and can discourage the patient or relative from discussing their feelings. When we first set up the clinic, a semi-structured interview was used which provided a framework for specific areas to discuss. Of late, the interview assessment form is used for audit purposes only and is completed after the interview.

Each component of the interview will now be discussed in more detail, in order of the main aims of the clinic in Table 10.5.

Table 10.5 Main aims of the follow-up clinic

- Patients and relatives to understand their critical illness and about their ICU stay
- Patients and relatives to gain information about rehabilitation after critical illness
- To provide advice and support for patients and relatives
- To identify any physical, psychological or social problems, and refer to appropriate specialities
- To promote a quality service. Feedback from patients and relatives will initiate changes in clinical practice
- To provide feedback of a patient's progress to ICU staff

Patient's critical illness and intensive care stay

The majority of intensive care patients remember little of their intensive care stay (Daffurn *et al.*, 1994). This lack of recall can lead to misconceptions and unrealistic expectations of themselves during their recovery (Griffiths *et al.*, 1996). Many patients do not know why it is taking some time to recover, which leads to anxieties, frustrations and psychological problems during their recovery. Information about their critical illness helps them to understand how ill they have been and to set realistic goals for their recovery.

The areas listed in Table 10.6 are discussed during the initial stages of the interview. The patient's reason for intensive care admission is explained, with an explanation of the significant ICU events. Some of this information may not be new to the patient or their relative, but certain areas may require clarification or questions answered. Any misunderstandings can be dealt with at this time. Whenever possible questions are answered in full, but occasionally the follow-up sister is unable to provide adequate information. In these cases, advice is sought from the appropriate professionals.

Table 10.6 Patient's critical illness and ICU stay

- Explanation of reason for ICU admission and significant events in ICU
- Clarification of points
- Answer questions
- Long-term health and prognosis
- Memories, delusions, nightmares, dreams
- Visit to ICU

Once a good rapport has been established, it is an opportunity to discuss their illness, prognosis and, with appropriate patients, their feelings about future admissions to ICU (for example patients with advanced respiratory disease). Some patients may feel they would not want to go through the experience again. Conversely, some would want to receive treatment, but medical staff have stated that further admission to ICU would be inappropriate. It is important to discuss these issues in a calm and open environment, where the patient can express his or her wishes. The patient's feelings about readmission to ICU are written in the medical notes, with the patient's agreement, and brought to the attention of their hospital consultant.

Patient's memories of ICU are varied and some examples are listed in Table 10.7. Some memories reflect the true events, but others are surreal or a distortion of reality. Any distorted memories are highlighted and, if possible, put into context.

Some patients have frightening memories of ICU; others cannot put their memories into perspective. We encourage patients and relatives to visit the unit,

Table 10.7 Patients' memories

- 'I felt the metal blade and the tube going into my throat, the room was full of people'.
- 'I would not close my eyes, as I was so frightened of the horrific nightmares'.
- 'I heard the nurse saying horrible things about my mother'.
- 'I felt like a leper'.
- 'Going to the ward was the worst day of my life'.
- 'Mouth swabs were truly wonderful'.
- 'It was torture hearing a can of coke being opened or seeing anyone have a drink'.

---

when they feel ready. The reality of seeing ICU is less scary than their images of the unit. After the initial apprehension, it can be beneficial to piece together events when prompted by noises, faces, voices, smells or the layout of the unit. Patients' comments regarding the return visit include: 'it explained certain memories and visions'; 'was not as awful as I had imagined or remembered'; 'it put it all into context'; 'it dispelled myths'; 'helped me close the book and to move forward'. Relatives have also found a return visit therapeutic in helping them come to terms with their experiences and to move on with their lives.

Dreams, nightmares, hallucinations and delusions have been a common problem for 70% of patients attending our clinic. Some examples are described in Table 10.8. For many, their experiences were vivid, real and terrifying. They often involved death, torture or violence.

An explanation of the possible causes of these experiences is discussed with the patient. These include the physiological effects of critical illness; the use of sedative and opiate drugs; disorientation; lack of differentiation between day and night; sleep deprivation and sensory overload (Campbell *et al.*, 1986). Patients greatly benefit from being told 'they are not going mad' and feel reassured that others have had similar experiences. The patients have these experiences during

Table 10.8 Patients' dreams or delusions

- 'A dead man in a coffin was in the next door room, and nurses were dancing around it with pink aprons on'.
- 'A man was trying to burn me to death'.
- 'There were dead people at the end of the unit, I was the next in line to go there'.
- 'I was in a boat, getting away from people out to kill me'.
- 'I needed to pull everything out, so I could bleed myself to death'.
- 'I was terrified, they were out to murder me and I had to get away'.

---

their ICU stay and occasionally on the ward, but the majority do not suffer with them at home. The memory of the experience remains clear in their mind and many find them difficult to forget. They often need to put them into context but this is usually very difficult. Some people remain distressed by their experiences and are unable to cope; these patients require referral to a clinical psychologist.

Rehabilitation information, advice and support

The majority of patients and relatives receive little information about rehabilitation after critical illness. General practitioners have limited experience in this field (Griffiths, 1992; Audit Commission, 1999) and hospital consultants have time constraints, which inhibit patients from receiving adequate advice about rehabilitation.

The follow-up appointment is an ideal opportunity to discuss recovery from critical illness and related issues, as listed in Table 10.9.

Table 10.9 Rehabilitation information

- Information and support
- Expectations and setting realistic goals
- Transition from the sick role
- Lifestyle changes

Information, support and explanation about recovery is essential, to assist the patient and their relatives during this very difficult time. This involves encouraging exercise, a healthy diet and activities to assist their recovery. Discussing expectations of both the patient and their relative and helping to set realistic goals also plays an important part in the interview. Talking about the transition from the sick role and, when appropriate, coming to terms with lifestyle changes, can be extremely beneficial. Some patients simply need reassurance that they will improve physically and psychologically, and return to their normal state of health. Rehabilitation is discussed in more detail in Chapter 11.

Identifying problems and referrals

Many of the patients attending the follow-up clinic have physical, psychological and social problems, either as a result of their critical illness or due to other underlying medical conditions. Relatives have also been through a very traumatic experience and some suffer psychological and social problems as a consequence of their experiences.

Table 10.10 Physical, psychological and social issues

- Respiratory and cardiovascular:
  Breathlessness, cough, sputum, wheeze, chest pain, palpitations, panic attacks

- Genitourinary:
  Frequency and pain during micturition, sex life and libido, menstruation

- Mobility:
  Walking/running, aids, stairs, joint stiffness, muscle weakness, getting in and out of a car, driving, housework, activities of daily living

- Eating:
  Weight loss or gain, diet, appetite changes, indigestion, bowel habits

- Central nervous system and senses:
  Dizziness, balance, vision, black outs, pins and needles, neuropathy, headaches

- Sleeping:
  Sleep pattern, insomnia, nightmares, night sedation

- Skin, hair and nails:
  Rashes, dryness, bruising, scarring, itching, hair loss, hair texture, weak nails, body image, general appearance

- Ear, nose and throat:
  Voice changes, tracheostomy site, tracheal stenosis, hearing

- Pain:
  When and where, interference with normal activities, scale of pain, medication

- Emotions:
  Tearfulness, mood swings, irritability, depression, anxiety, nervousness, confidence, concentration, nightmares, delusions, daily activities, perceptions of health

- Social changes:
  Lifestyle changes, role in family, relationships, change in family dynamics, social activities, financial problems, work

---

The patient and their relative are informally assessed at the follow-up appointment. We discuss physical, psychological and social health issues (including current treatment), as shown in Table 10.10. The physical issues relate to the patient's health, the psychological and social issues are discussed with reference to the patient and their relative.

Good communication and interpersonal skills are required to obtain accurate information and requirement for appropriate referral. To confirm our assessment of the person, we ask the patient and their relative to complete, individually, the hospital anxiety and depression (HAD) scale (Zigmond and Snaith, 1983) and the

Table 10.11 Common physical problems

- Weakness
- Weight loss
- Fatigue
- Painful joints
- Peripheral neuropathy
- Poor appetite
- Voice and taste changes
- Insomnia
- Impotence
- Skin and nail changes
- Hair loss
- Pruritus
- Amenorrhoea

Short form 36 (UK version) health survey (Ware, 1992). Both forms have been helpful in providing an indication of psychological health status and in confirming a requirement for referral.

Common problems we have seen at our clinic are summarized in Tables 10.11 and 10.12. The causes of these problems and appropriate treatment are discussed in more detail in other chapters of this book.

The follow-up sister usually refers the patient or relative directly to the appropriate speciality. In some cases, a discussion with the intensive care consultant is necessary for advice on appropriate referral. Some of the common referrals are listed in Table 10.13.

If the patient or a relative requires referral for a specific problem, it is discussed with them and the plan mutually agreed. This is essential for

Table 10.12 Common psychological and social problems

- Depression
- Anxiety
- Panic attacks
- Post-traumatic stress disorder
- Guilt
- Lack of confidence
- Loss of libido
- Irritability and intolerance
- Poor memory and concentration
- Social isolation
- Marital difficulties
- Financial difficulties

Table 10.13 Common referrals

- Physician
- Surgeon
- Counsellor
- Clinical psychologist
- Physiotherapist
- General practitioner
- Dermatologist
- Psychosexual counsellor
- ENT
- Dietician
- Neurologist
- Infection control and microbiologist

---

psychological problems; the person needs some insight into their problem and agrees to be referred for professional help.

Hospital consultants accept referrals from the clinic and are contacted by telephone, e-mail or letter, depending on the urgency of the specific problem. For example, Mr D is a 70-year-old man, who was in ICU for 14 days after a routine abdominal aortic aneurysm repair. During his ICU stay, he was diagnosed with ischaemic heart disease and was seen by a cardiologist. After leaving ICU, Mr F was discharged to general medical ward and then home. At his ICU follow-up appointment, Mr F explained about his increasing angina attacks. He experienced the attacks two or three times a day, for which he was taking GTN spray. He had told the general physician about this, at his routine outpatient appointment. The follow-up sister telephoned Mr F's GP to discuss his problem, and Mr F went to see his GP the same day. The follow-up sister also sent a referral letter to the cardiologist.

After each clinic consultation, the follow-up sister completes the assessment form and writes a comprehensive summary of the interview. This includes identifying problems and referrals required, together with the patient and relatives comments about their ICU care. This report is confidential, and is filed for future appointments and for data collection purposes.

Changes in clinical practice and promoting a quality service

The follow-up clinic has provided an effective evaluation of nursing and medical practices on our ICU. The feedback from patients and relatives about their experiences on ICU has initiated changes in clinical practice. Their comments have been invaluable and now provide a framework for issues relating to clinical governance (Crinson, 1999). The changes in clinical practice as a result of this feedback must be placed in perspective; 98% of the people attending the clinic believed their ICU care to be excellent, but the areas of change have made an improvement to the overall service provided. Some practice developments include:

- Staff have drinks away from the patients' bed space, as patients have commented 'it was torture to watch staff drinking'.
- Clocks and white boards are visible at each patient's bed space, to promote patient orientation.
- The purchase of new rubbish bins, as the noise of previous bin lids closing broke patients' sleep.
- Improving information for patients with MRSA, following their feedback about loneliness, isolation and 'how they felt like a leper'.
- A change of our synthetic colloid policy after an investigation into severe itching. At our clinic, 30% of patients complained of pruritus, which initiated a larger audit and a change of policy (Sharland et al., 1999).
- The publication of an 'After intensive care booklet' for patients and relatives (who have been in ICU for more than 4 days). All ICU patients and relatives receive a discharge information sheet. These were initiated by patients' comments about the 'first day on the ward was the worst day of my whole life'.
- Changes in the ICU discharge process to improve continuity of patient care and to help the transition from ICU to the ward. This includes a new ICU discharge transfer form.
- A medical ICU discharge summary form has been produced to promote continuity of medical care, to optimize treatment and prevent errors in clinical practice.
- Discharge letters to the patient's GP are now sent on the patient's discharge from ICU.
- The ICU follow-up sister visits former ICU patients on the ward, as a result of patients' comments about their ward experiences.
- Changes in staff attitudes and their nursing care, as a result of greater awareness of patient and relatives' experiences of ICU. Examples include: reducing noise levels, encouraging sleep with a normal day-night cycle, repetition of information, regular mouth care and a greater use of communication aids.

Feedback to ICU staff

A brief summary is written after each follow-up interview and is available for feedback to all the unit staff. Any personal or sensitive information is not included in this report.

Comments from patients and relatives have helped to promote the continuation of good clinical practice. For example, the relatives found the staff caring, capable and delivered a high quality service. They valued honest information with no false hope, regular condition updates, understanding and empathy from all staff members. It is beneficial for staff to be aware of their good practice and for it to be acknowledged. This can encourage staff morale and a good working environment, which will reflect on staff retention and recruitment.

Staff teaching sessions are an essential part of the follow-up sister's role. They provide an opportunity for staff education and to disseminate information gleaned from the follow-up clinic. It has been well documented that 'it is important to give ICU staff the chance to understand the process of recovery from critical illness, and to examine the effects on patients of their own practice' (Jones *et al.*, 1994).

Audit and evaluation of the follow-up service

Every patient and their relative has a follow-up clinic evaluation form, the HAD scale (Zigmond and Snaith, 1983) and the UK Short form 36 health survey (Ware, 1992), to complete at home. The questionnaires are confidential and returned by post. The ICU follow-up sister completes the interview assessment form after each consultation. The clinic evaluation form and assessment form are used for audit purposes to evaluate the effectiveness of the clinic.

Recently, we have been auditing the requirement for a physiotherapy service, specifically for former ICU patients. At present, the follow-up sister refers a patient to the hospital outpatient physiotherapist or to their local health centre. The results of the audit show that ICU survivors experience varying degrees of physical limitation following discharge from hospital. There is a need for early physiotherapy input by an experienced physiotherapist, which would lead to an overall improvement in physical and psychological well-being. As a result of the audit, we hope to include a physiotherapy service into our future business plan proposal.

Further audit and research are planned for the future to help evaluate and improve our ICU services.

Ward visits

Patients' and relatives' comments about their ward experiences initiated the expansion of our service. It now includes regular ward visits to former ICU patients from the ICU follow-up sister and our newly established critical care outreach team. The ICU follow-up sister routinely visits patients who were in ICU for more than 4 days. On returning to the ward, patients and relatives understandably feel vulnerable, insecure and anxious. The sudden lack of nursing staff and technical equipment around their bed area causes some of this anxiety. They need help to reduce the stress associated with this experience.

The follow-up sister visits patients and relatives regularly, up to their discharge home. The outreach team focuses on the patient's acute care problems and will discharge them from their care when the patient's condition is stable.

During the ward visit, the follow-up sister discusses the patient's ICU stay, if the timing is appropriate. The visit also provides an opportunity to get to know the patient and their relatives, and to identify any long-term health problems. The ICU discharge booklet is given to them, which contains information for patients and relatives about ICU discharge, together with advice regarding recovery and describes possible problems. The ICU follow-up helpline is explained to patients and relatives. The helpline is not a 24-hour service; an answer machine is available, and the follow-up sister returns calls during daytime working hours.

The ward visit encourages patients and relatives to begin preparation for their recovery from critical illness, with the reassurance of support and advice from the ICU follow-up sister.

The future

The development and expansion of the follow-up service is planned for the future. A business plan proposal is required to increase resources and secure funding for a designated clinical psychologist, counsellor and physiotherapist. We would also like to expand the service to include all our ICU patients and relatives, and those from other hospitals where this facility is not available.

Another development opportunity involves running a comprehensive rehabilitation programme, with similarities to the cardiac rehabilitation programme. The intensive care recovery manual (Jones, 1998) appears to be an effective tool to aid patients and relatives in their recovery and would be very beneficial for some of our patients.

Feedback to GPs requires improvement and development, to increase their awareness of the short- and long-term effects of critical illness on patients and their relatives. Working more closely with GPs will promote seamless care from hospital to the community, which will ultimately impact on the patient's recovery.

Further research, audit and practice development will be both interesting and essential in this exciting area, to improve outcomes and quality of life of ICU survivors and their relatives. Networking and sharing ideas with other follow-up services may be a good way forward, to enable these ideas to become reality.

In conclusion

The setting up of a nurse-led clinic is achievable with minimal resources. An experienced ICU nurse with enthusiasm and interest in this area is ideally suited to run this clinic. The ability to organize a therapeutic interview and to know when to ask for advice are essential qualities for this role. An effective follow-up service depends on the support of the intensive care multidisciplinary team and other healthcare professionals.

Patients and relatives benefit from this invaluable service. ICU follow-up care improves the quality of recovery from critical illness and has an impact on the quality of life of former ICU patients and their relatives. The findings from our follow-up clinic have acknowledged existing good practice and identified areas for clinical improvement. The changes in practice have enhanced the quality of nursing and medical care for ICU patients and relatives. Further research and audit will be fundamental for the future development of intensive care aftercare.

A follow-up service is essential to promote a quality service for patients and relatives, both during and after their intensive care stay.

References

Audit commission. *Critical to Success. The place of efficient and effective critical care services within the acute hospital.* Audit Commission, London: October 1999.

Campbell IT, Minors DS, Waterhouse JM Are circadian rhythms important in intensive care? *Intensive Care Nursing* 1986; **1**,144–50.

Compton P Critical illness and intensive care: what it means to the client. *Critical Care Nurse* 1991; **11**, 50–6.

Crinson I Clinical governance: the new NHS, new responsibilities? *British Journal of Nursing* 1999; **7**, 449–53.

Daffurn K, Bishop GF, Hillman KM, Bauman A Problems following discharge after intensive care. *Intensive and Critical Care Nursing* 1994; **10**, 244–51.

Department of Health *Comprehensive Critical Care. A review of adult critical care services.* HMSO, London: 2000.

Griffiths RD Development of normal indices of recovery from critical illness. In: (Rennie MJ, ed.) *Intensive Care Britain.* Greycote Publishing, London: 1992, pp 134–7.

Griffiths RD, Jones C, Macmillan RR Where is the harm in not knowing? Care after intensive care. *Clinical Intensive Care* 1996; **7**, 144–5.

Hackman JR, Lawler EE Employee reactions to job characteristics. *Journal of Applied Psychology Monograph* 1971; **3**, 259–86.

Jones C *Intensive Care Recovery Manual.* Whiston Hospital, 1998.

Jones C, Humphris GM, Griffiths RD Psychological morbidity following critical illness – the rationale for care after intensive care. *Clinical Intensive Care* 1998; **9**, 199–205.

Jones C, Macmillan RR, Griffiths RD Providing psychological support for patients after critical illness. *Clinical Intensive Care* 1994; **5**, 176–9.

Ley P, Spelman MS Communications in an out-patient setting. *British Journal of the Society of Clinical Psychology* 1965; **4**, 114–16.

Myerscough PR *Talking with Patients.* Oxford Medical Publications, Oxford: 1992, pp 37–44.

Ramsey R Invited review: Post-traumatic stress disorder; a new clinical entity? *Journal of Psychosomatic Research* 1990; **34**, 355–65.

Sharland C, Huggett A, Nielsen M Persistent pruritus after hydroxyethyl starch (HES) infusions in critically ill patients. *Critical Care* 1999; **3**(suppl 1), 150.

Tschudin V *Counselling Skills for Nurses*. Baillière Tindall, London: 1995, pp 68–91.

Ware J, Sherbourne C The MOS 36-Item Short-Form Health Survey 1: conceptual framework and item selection. *Medical Care* 1992; **30**, 473–83.

Zigmond AS, Snaith RP The Hospital Anxiety and Depression Scale. *Acta Psychiatrica Scandinavica* 1983; **67**, 361–70.

Rehabilitation after critical illness

Christina Jones and Richard D. Griffiths

Introduction

Intensive care unit (ICU) patients face a common core of physical and psychological problems during the recovery period, despite differing presenting diagnoses. Muscle wasting and profound weakness are common and physical recovery is slow, measured in months rather than weeks (Jones and Griffiths, 2000). Patients often display high levels of psychological distress (Jones et al., 1998). Research into rehabilitation following critical illness is limited, with a focus on pulmonary rehabilitation (Nava and Ambrosino, 2000).

Background

Rehabilitation studies have shown that exercise regimens and psychological intervention programmes have proved to be effective in aiding recovery and coping behaviour in patients with widely differing diagnoses, e.g. chronic obstructive pulmonary disease (Kaplan et al., 1995), chronic fatigue syndrome (Fulcher and White, 1997) and myocardial infarction patients (Sandler et al., 1999).

Pulmonary rehabilitation

In a study of mild to severe chronic obstructive pulmonary disease (COPD), 119 patients were randomized to receive either rehabilitation or health education. Rehabilitation consisted of exercise training, coping strategies, information on

COPD and weekly psychosocial support groups over 8 weeks, and then monthly sessions for 1 year. Rehabilitation improved the patients' exercise tolerance and symptoms compared to the control patients. However, this difference tended to decrease with time and was absent by the 4-year follow-up (Ries *et al.*, 1992).

Carrieri-Kohlman *et al.* (1993) found that desensitization, through guided mastery, to situations that would normally cause COPD patients to panic helps these patients to cope with their breathlessness.

Patients suffering from severe impairment of ventilation due to non-obstructive pulmonary disease, for example pneumonia or adult respiratory distress syndrome, can benefit from pulmonary rehabilitation. This type of patient has usually spent quite a time in ICU and while dyspnoea causes exercise limitation, muscle wasting may exacerbate this. While these patients only formed 10% of the patient population attending the pulmonary rehabilitation programme reported by Novitch and Thomas (1993), they felt that these patients show a similar improvement in exercise tolerance with rehabilitation as those suffering from chronic obstructive pulmonary disease.

Rehabilitation post-myocardial infarction

Rehabilitation programmes for myocardial infarction patients initially were purely exercise based. These programmes showed a 20% reduction in overall mortality. The addition of relaxation training and breathing exercises improves this to 50% (Van Dixhoorn *et al.*, 1989). A home-based exercise programme has been found to be as effective as a hospital-based one and, in fact, may improve compliance due to the habit of exercise being developed and maintained within the home (O'Rourke *et al.*, 1990). Rehabilitation exercise programmes alone have also been shown to have a moderate beneficial effect on anxiety and depression levels in coronary patients (Kugler *et al.*, 1994). In addition, written advice on smoking cessation in myocardial infarction patients has been shown to result in a high rate of cessation (69%) at 1 year (Moreno *et al.*, 2000). It has been suggested that rehabilitation programmes giving specific anti-smoking advice may be effective in aiding smoking cessation and that exercise may also aid smoking cessation (Ussher *et al.*, 2000). This is an important issue for patients recovering from ICU. The lung damage that results from illnesses such as pneumonia or adult respiratory distress syndrome will not be given a chance to recover if patients return to smoking post-ICU.

Relatives of myocardial infarction patients struggle to cope with the patients' illness (Hentinen, 1983). Most of the family want information about caring for the patient when they come home. This is an issue echoed by relatives of ICU patients.

It might be expected then that ICU patients might benefit from a rehabilitation programme following critical illness. However, there are differences between ICU patients and also any other patient group, the main one being the memory problems for the period of acute illness that these patients experience (see Chapter 2). ICU patients' psychological recovery may be complicated by memories from the period of critical illness (Schelling *et al.*, 1998; Jones *et al.*, 2001a).

ICU rehabilitation manual

The ICU rehabilitation manual was developed to include information and practical advice on common problems likely to be encountered by ICU patients during their recovery. The scarcity of research into rehabilitation in ICU patients led to the examination of literature published in similar fields, such as the rehabilitation of myocardial infarction patients and the problems their relatives face during the convalescent period. Lewin *et al.* (1992) showed a 50% reduction in anxiety levels with myocardial infarction patients using a self-help rehabilitation booklet, the *Hearts Manual*, designed to reduce psychological distress and encourage physical recovery using graded exercises.

The ICU manual was designed from the information gained from years of following-up patients. Using the layout of the Hearts Manual the ICU rehabilitation manual was devided into three separate books.

Book 1 is made up of 6 weekly parts with an exercise record, fitness plan and information. The information covers such problems as the possible physical sequelae of critical illness, e.g. muscle wasting, weakness, hair loss, taste changes and appetite loss; the possible psychosocial sequelae, e.g. marital friction or overprotective family; and the psychological sequelae, e.g. panic attacks, phobias, anxiety and depression. There is also information to emphasize the normality of these reactions after severe stress. In addition, there is more general advice on areas such as stress management and anxiety, relaxation, getting back their normal fitness level, eating well and sexual problems after major illness. The importance of quitting smoking following critical illness is emphasized in weeks 1, 3 and 6 of the manual, with practical advice being provided and two successful patient stories included as encouragement.

An important principle of the design was that the educational programme should be patient-centred. Patients are expected to take responsibility for their own health. So, in addition to information, patients are asked to reflect and think about themselves through quizzes. This ensures that the programme is relevant to the widest possible range of patients as the quizzes lead patients on to extra sections in the second half of the manual where they can find more information about an individual problem.

Book 2 contains more detailed self-help advice on a wide range of problems. First, dealing with psychological problems, such as panic attacks, phobias, anxiety and depression and information on when and how to turn to professional help through their GP and what is realistically available. Secondly, advice is given on supplementing nutrition if the appetite is poor and which foods are important to eat. Thirdly, common-sense advice on how to overcome sexual problems after major illness. Other miscellaneous areas covered are living alone, medicines, and stress in marriage. Instructions in section 1 of the manual direct patients to read particular pages in section 2, which are relevant to their individual needs.

Book 3 was developed in discussion with a senior physiotherapist (Marie Swinfield) with experience in rehabilitation. This consists of a graded exercise programme, but its design needed a new approach because of the heterogeneous nature of the ICU population. In addition to a large age range, patients may have disabilities left after ICU from injuries due to trauma or have already a considerable degree of chronic ill-health before admission. One set of exercises would simply not be able to cope with this wide range. To help patients to regain a sense of control over their health it was felt that the exercise programme should also be patient directed with only the body areas to be exercised prescribed. Ratings of perceived exertion (RPE) provide a very simple tool. A number of studies have shown that RPE can be used successfully in a variety of populations (Dunbar *et al.*, 1992; Eakin *et al.*, 1992; Dishman, 1994). Bearing in mind the heterogeneous ICU population, with the wide variety of physical problems and fitness levels, the use of RPE, backed up with advice on what exercises to select and when to stop exercising, seemed the most suitable tool in the circumstances.

Patients are instructed to choose a set number of exercises and then use the Borg Exertional scale (Borg, 1982) to ensure that they exercise within a specified exertional difficulty. The duration of each exercise to be practised or the number of repetitions is under the patients' control. They are instructed to increase or decrease the number of repetitions themselves to bring the exercise into the right range of exertion. For the arm exercises, small weights are recommended, e.g. sugar or salt weighed into a plastic bag and the top of the bag knotted. Advice is given to ensure that patients do not use inappropriately heavy weights, again using the Borg Exertional scale.

Rehabilitation study

Using a block randomized, controlled design, blind at follow-up, routine ICU follow-up was compared with routine follow-up plus a 6 weeks self-help rehabilitation programme. Physical and psychological recovery was assessed at 2 and 6 months post-ICU. To examine the influence of delusional memories of hallucinations or paranoid delusions from ICU on psychological distress the impact of memories of ICU on psychological recovery was also assessed in a proportion of the patients.

The study ran over 2 years and patients were recruited at three hospitals, Whiston Hospital, Merseyside (W), Manchester Royal Infirmary (M) and Royal Berkshire Hospital, Reading (R) (Jones *et al.*, 2001b).

Physical and psychological measures used to test the rehabilitation manual

To assess physical and psychological recovery, evaluations took place at 2 weeks, and 2 and 6 months post-ICU discharge. A separate researcher, who was not aware of which group the patient was in, conducted the follow-up. Trait anxiety was assessed at recruitment using the Spielberger's State-trait Anxiety Inventory (STAI) (Spielberger *et al.*, 1970). Anxiety and depression scores were recorded using the Hospital Anxiety and Depression Scale (Zigmond and Snaith, 1983) (HAD). The Impact of Events Scale (IES) was used at 8 weeks and 6 months to assess PTSD-related symptoms (Horowitz *et al.*, 1979). Memory for the time on ICU was assessed using the ICU Memory Tool (Jones *et al.*, 2000). The Short form health survey (SF-36) physical function scores was used to assess physical recovery at 2 and 6 months (Ware, 1992). Patients also completed the SF-36 at recruitment to the study but were asked about their pre-morbid health in the 6 months before admission to ICU.

The ICU rehabilitation manual contains advice on the importance of giving up smoking. There has been little research on smoking cessation post-critical illness. Smokers make up a high percentage of patients admitted to intensive care (ICU) for community-acquired pneumonia (Ortqvist *et al.*, 1985) and postoperative complications. Stopping smoking should be one message that should be clearly given to recovering intensive care (ICU) patients. The recovery period provides an important opportunity for patients to quit smoking as the time on the ICU of sedation and ventilation allows patients to start nicotine withdrawal. Written advice on smoking cessation in other patient groups, such as myocardial infarction, has been shown to result in a high quit rate (69%) at one year. Furthermore, rehabilitation programmes giving specific anti-smoking advice are effective in aiding smoking cessation in other patient groups (Dinnes, 1998). This is an important issue for many patients recovering after ICU. The recovery of lung damage resulting from illnesses such as pneumonia or adult respiratory distress syndrome may be compromised if the patient continues to damage their lungs by smoking post-ICU. For this reason, in a proportion of patients the impact of the manual on smoking cessation was assessed.

Patients in the treatment group were introduced to the ICU rehabilitation manual, with a close relative or friend present. Work with myocardial infarction patients has shown that including relatives in the provision of information increases patient compliance with advice (Van Elderen-van Kemenade *et al.*, 1994).

Physical recovery

One hundred and twenty-six patients were recruited across the three study centres. At 6 months, 58/69 (84%) interventions patients and 44/57 (77%)

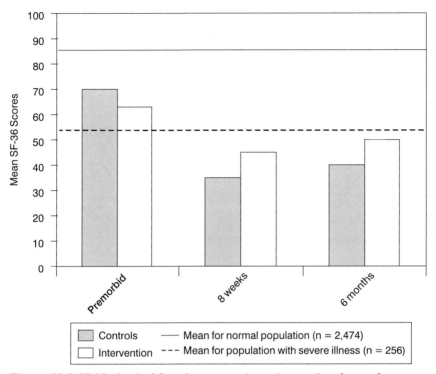

Figure 11.1 SF-36 physical function scores (mean) over time by study group

controls completed the study. Ten patients died (5 intervention, 5 controls) before 6 month follow-up.

Intervention patients seemed to be recovering faster as they showed significantly higher SF-36 physical function scores at 8 weeks and 6 months than control patients ($P = 0.006$) (Figure 11.1).

Smoking cessation

Thirty-one intervention and 30 control patients were recruited at Whiston Hospital and a record of smoking habits prior to ICU admission made; 20/31 intervention patients and 16/30 control patients were smokers pre-ICU admission. At the 8 week follow-up, two patients (10%) in the intervention groups had resumed smoking compared with five (31%) in the control group. This effect was more marked at the 6 month follow-up, with three (15%) of the intervention patients returning to smoking and 10 (62%) in the control group ($P = 0.006$). This therapy therefore gave a reduction in smoking risk of 89% (CI 36–98%), particularly important as one wishes to promote the healing of damaged lungs.

There was no difference in anxiety, depression or PTSD-related symptoms at 6 months between patients who continued to smoke and those who quit.

Psychological recovery

Using the cut-off of > 11 on the HAD scale as indicating depression, at 8 weeks a smaller percentage of intervention patients were depressed, 12% versus 25%, but this did not reach statistical significance ($P = 0.066$). At 6 months the rate of depression in the two study groups was the same, 10% in the intervention group and 12% in control patients.

There was no difference in the incidence of anxiety between the two study groups, either at 8 weeks or 6 months. The incidence of anxiety remained quite high at 33% in both groups at 6 months.

Symptoms of PTSD were considerably lower in the intervention patients at 8 weeks ($P = 0.026$), but there was no difference at 6 months.

Effect of delusional memories

Fifty-two patients recruited to the study at Whiston Hospital were asked about the presence of delusional memories from ICU. Those patients who could recall delusional memories had higher HAD anxiety scores at 8 weeks and 6 months than those without delusional memories ($P < 0.0001$; $P < 0.001$ respectively). Similarly IES scores, indicating symptoms of PTSD, were higher in both study groups for those patients recalling delusional memories at 6 months than those without delusional memories (Figure 11.2).

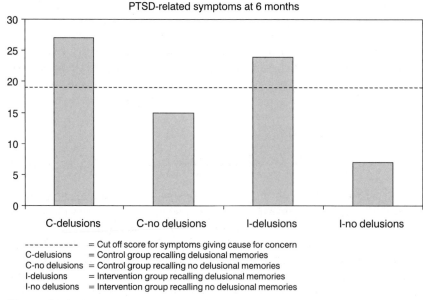

Figure 11.2 Mean Impact of Events Scale scores by study group and recall of delusional memories from ICU at 6 months post-ICU

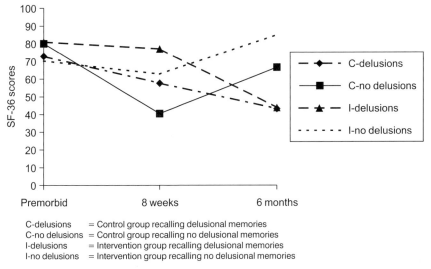

C-delusions   = Control group recalling delusional memories
C-no delusions = Control group recalling no delusional memories
I-delusions   = Intervention group recalling delusional memories
I-no delusions = Intervention group recalling no delusional memories

Figure 11.3 Comparison of SF-36 emotional role scores by study group and recall of delusional memories

Horowitz (1986) suggested a score of > 19 on the IES as indicating a level of PTSD-related symptoms that was a cause for concern. Fifty-two (51%) of the 102 study patients scored in this range at 6 months post-ICU. This was equally divided between the study groups, 21/44 (48%) control, 31/58 (53%) intervention patients. When those patients with data on recall of delusional memories on ICU were examined, 21 of 35 (60%) patients with delusional memories scored > 19 and five of 18 (28%) without such memories at 6 months post-ICU ($P = 0.028$).

A similar pattern was seen with the SF-36 Emotional Role scores when recall of delusional memories in ICU was examined. Those patients recalling delusional memories, regardless of study group, were more likely to be scoring highly for psychological distress than those without such recall (Figure 11.3).

Discussion

The ICU rehabilitation package proved to be successful in significantly aiding physical function recovery and there was a suggestion also that the rate of depression was reduced with a halving of the incidence at 8 weeks. These results are similar to those found in myocardial patients (Fulcher and White, 1997). In addition, patients receiving the rehabilitation package were much less likely to return to smoking after discharge from ICU than the control patients. This was despite the control patients receiving verbal encouragement to quit smoking during the recovery period. There is insufficient evidence to determine whether the smoking cessation advice in the ICU rehabilitation package or the whole package in general was responsible for the high quit rate. It has been reported that exercise may aid smoking cessation. This may mean that it is not simply the smoking cessation advice in the ICU rehabilitation manual that is having an effect on whether patients return to smoking, but also the provision of an exercise programme. Certainly the combination of life-threatening illness and structured written advice on stopping smoking seems to result in high rates of cessation.

The ICU rehabilitation manual, however, did not have the same effect on reducing anxiety rates as seen using a self-directed rehabilitation package with myocardial infarction patients. High anxiety scores were particularly seen in patients recalling delusional memories, regardless of study group. The fact that > 30% of all the patients on the study were anxious at 6 months shows that this is a significant problem and needs to be addressed. This is despite the rehabilitation package containing information on coping strategies that have been shown to break the worry/anxiety cycle, such as recognition of symptoms to aid self-awareness, relaxation and challenging the thoughts causing anxiety (Stern and Drummond, 1991). A similar pattern was also seen with PTSD-related symptoms; 51% of all the patients completing the study scored above the cut-off of 19 at 6 months. This is a very high incidence of PTSD-related symptoms and is a real cause for concern. In common with the HAD anxiety scores the patients who had the highest IES scores were those patients recalling delusional memories from ICU in both study groups.

The quality of cognitive processing at the time of the traumatic event seems to be important in the development of PTSD. Those reporting confusion and being overwhelmed at the time of the traumatic situation seem to be more likely to suffer from chronic PTSD (Ehlers and Clark, 2000). One of the problems with the delusional memories recalled by ICU patients is that these are reported as being very realistic, vivid and frightening. If factual memories can also be recalled patients can possibly make sense of the delusional memories by reasoning that they are due to their illness and the treatment they received. These patients know that the illness happened to them rather than having to be told later.

Why ICU patients vary so widely in their recall of ICU is not clear. Certainly those patients with high trait anxiety scores were more likely to recall delusional memories and go on to develop high levels of PTSD-related symptoms at 8 weeks post-ICU (Jones et al., 2001a). This agrees with studies of victims of other types of traumatizing events where one predisposing factor for chronic PTSD has been shown to be an anxiety-prone personality. Perhaps patients with high trait anxiety have a greater propensity to assess their surrounding as hostile and so are more likely to develop hallucinations and paranoid delusions in ambiguous situations such as ICU, particularly when their cognition is affected by illness and sedative medication. This is supported by work in elderly individuals, which suggests that anxiety-proneness is linked to the development of delirium in highly ambiguous or stressful situations.

The psychological problems of patients that appear to be caused by the presence of delusional memories of ICU strongly indicate the need for this group to receive special attention in rehabilitation research. What the ICU rehabilitation manual clearly is not addressing are the worries and concerns of those patients who have delusional memories from their time on ICU. While some mention was made in the ICU rehabilitation manual of nightmares, hallucinations and delusions and how frightening and realistic they can be, no specific information was given on the normality of PTSD-related symptoms etc. This could be added to the programme, however, with such a high rate of PTSD-related symptoms it is difficult to imagine such an intervention having more than a moderate impact. There is perhaps a role here for more formal counselling or the design of a specific psychological intervention.

Despite this, the results suggest that a rehabilitation package is a useful initial intervention to aid physical and psychological recovery. However, rehabilitation would have to be combined with screening for delusional memories as it is likely that these patients would need further psychological intervention.

References

Borg GAV Psychophysical basis of perceived exertion. *Medical Science Sports Exercise* 1982; **14**(5), 377–81.

Carrieri-Kohlman V, Douglas MK, Gormley JM, Stulburg MS Desensitization and guided mastery: treatment approaches for the management of dyspnoea. *Heart and Lung* 1993; **22**(3), 226–34.

Dinnes J Cardiac rehabilitation. *Nursing Times* 1998; **94**(38), 50–2.

Dishman RK Prescribing exercise intensity for healthy adults using perceived exertion. *Medical Science Sports Exercise* 1994; **26**(9), 1087–94.

Dunbar CC, Robertson RJ, Baun R *et al*. The validation of regulating exercise intensity by ratings of perceived exertion. *Medical Science Sports Exercise* 1992; **24**(1), 94–9.

Eakin BL, Finta KM, Serwer GA, Beekman RH Perceived exertion and exercise intensity in children with and without structural heart defeats. *Journal of Paediatrics* 1992; **120**, 90–3.

Ehlers A, Clark DM A cognitive model of posttraumatic stress disorder. *Behavioural Research and Therapy* 2000; **38**, 319–45

Fulcher KY, White PD Randomised controlled trial of graded exercise in patients with chronic fatigue syndrome. *British Medical Journal* 1997; **314**, 1647–52.

Hentinen M Need for instruction and support of the wives of patients with myocardial infarction. *Journal of Advanced Nursing* 1983; **8**, 519–24.

Horowitz M, Wilner N, Alvarez W. Impact of events scale: a measure of subjective stress. *Psychosomatic Medicine* 1979; **41**(3), 209–18.

Horowitz M. *'Dosing' of trauma: Stress Response Syndromes*. Jason Aronson, Northvale, New Jersey: 1986.

Jones C, Griffiths RD Identifying post intensive care patients who may need physical rehabilitation. *Clinical Intensive Care* 2000; **11**(1), 35–8.

Jones C, Griffiths RD, Humphris G, Skirrow PM Memory, delusions and the development of acute post traumatic stress disorder-related symptoms after intensive care. *Critical Care Medicine* 2001a; **29**(3), 573–80.

Jones C, Humphris GM, Griffiths RD Psychological morbidity following critical illness – the rationale for care after intensive care. *Clinical Intensive Care* 1998; **9**, 199–205.

Jones C, Humphris G, Griffiths RD Preliminary validation of the ICUM tool: a tool for assessing memory of the intensive care experience. *Clinical Intensive Care* 2000; **11**(5), 251–5.

Jones C, Skirrow P, Griffiths RD *et al.* Rehabilitation after critical illness: a randomised, controlled trial. *British Journal of Anaesthesia* 2001b; **87**(2), 330.

Kaplan RAL, Limberg TM, Prewitt LM Effects of pulmonary rehabilitation on physiologic and psychosocial outcomes in patients with chronic obstructive pulmonary disease. *Annals of Internal Medicine* 1995; **122**, 823–32.

Kugler J, Seelbach H, Krüskernper GM Effects of rehabilitation exercise programmes on anxiety and depression in coronary patients: A meta-analysis. *British Journal of Clinical Psychology* 1994; **33**, 401–10.

Lewin B, Robertson IH, Cay EL, Irving JB, Campbell M Effects of self-help with post-myocardial infarction rehabilitation on psychological adjustment and use of health services. *Lancet* 1992; **339**, 1036–40.

Moreno OA, Ochoa GFJ, Ramalle-Gomara E, Saralegui RI, Fernandez EMV, Quintana DM Eficacia de una intervencion para dejar de fumar en pacientes con infarcto de miocardio. *Medicini Clinicia* 2000; **114**(6), 209–10.

Nava S, Ambrosino N Rehabilitation in the ICU: the European Phoenix. *Intensive Care Medicine* 2000: **26**, 841–4.

Novitch RS, Thomas HM Rehabilitation of patients with chronic ventilatory limitation from nonobstructive lung diseases. In (Casaburi R, Petty TL, eds) *Principles and Practice of Pulmonary Rehabilitation*. WB Saunders Company, Philadelphia: 1993, pp 416–23.

O'Rourke A, Levin B, Whitecross S The effects of physical exercise training and cardiac education on levels of anxiety and depression in the rehabilitation of coronary artery by-pass patients. *Intern Disability Studies* 1990; **12**, 104–6.

Ortqvist A, Sterner G, Nilsson JA Severe community-acquired pneumonia: factors influencing need of intensive care treatment and prognosis. *Scandinavian Journal of Infectious Diseases* 1985; **17**(4), 377–86.

Ries AL, Kaplan RM, Limberg TM, Prewitt LM Effects of pulmonary rehabilitation on physiological and psychosocial outcomes in patients with chronic obstructive pulmonary disease. *Annals of Internal Medicine* 1992; **122**, 823–32.

Sandler DA, Sandler G, Benison D, Wheatcroft S, Leakey P, Blair A Psychological and physical benefits of an exercise-based cardiac rehabilitation programme for patients recovering from a first MI. *British Journal of Cardiology* 1999; **6**(2), 102–12.

Schelling G, Stoll C, Meier M *et al.* Health-related quality of life and posttraumatic stress disorder in survivors of adult respiratory distress syndrome. *Critical Care Medicine* 1998; **26**, 651–9.

Spielberger CD, Gorsuch RL, Lushene R *State-trait Anxiety Inventory Manual*. Consulting Psychologists Press, Palo Alto, California: 1970.

Stern R, Drummond L *The Practice of Behavioural and Cognitive Psychotherapy*. Cambridge University Press, Cambridge: 1991.

Ussher MH, Taylor AH, West R, McEwen A Does exercise aid smoking cessation? A systematic review. *Addiction* 2000; **95**(2), 199–208.

Van Dixhoorn J, Duivenvoorden HJ, Staai HA Physical training and relaxation therapy in cardiac rehabilitation assessed through a composite criterion for training outcome. *American Heart Journal* 1989; **118**, 545–52.

Van Elderen-van Kemenade T, Maes S, van den Broek Y Effects of a health education programme with telephone follow-up during cardiac rehabilitation. *British Journal of Clinical Psychology* 1994; **33**, 367–78.

Ware JE, Sherbourne CD The MOS 36-item Short-Form Health Survey (SF-36). I. Conceptual framework and item selection. *Medical Care* 1992; **30**(6), 473–83.

Zigmond AS, Snaith RP The Hospital Anxiety and Depression Scale. *Acta Psychiatrica Scandinavica* 1983; **67**, 361–70.

Patient diaries in ICU

Carl Backmän

Introduction

Five years ago, in our ICU in Norrköping, Sweden, we started a group made up of five people who thought it would be interesting to show those patients who had been on the ventilator or been sedated for a long time what had happened to them. This was because many patients told us that they did not remember anything.

It was almost impossible to explain to these patients when they came back to see us or if we met them in normal life exactly what had happened to them. The relatives would recognize us but the patients did not, and the family would say, 'tell him how ill he has been, he does not believe us when we try to explain'. The patients often felt that they could not trust what the relatives said because they did not really understand the equipment used and the treatment. Some of the staff and even the relatives could not understand why the patients wanted to know what they had gone through; why could the patient not just stop thinking about it and concentrate on getting better?

The group thought that if we gave such patients a realistic description of their time in ICU, they might be a little less confused about what had happened, although we were not sure. To do this we decided to keep diaries of individual patient's ICU stays. This we hoped would let them come to terms with what they have gone through.

Method

A regular pocket-sized notebook was used to make the diaries and standard sets of rules for writing were followed.

Rules for writing in the diary

- Check with the patient or their relatives that they would like a diary to be kept and that they agree to photographs being taken. Inform them about the concept behind the diary and its importance (this means that if a patient is being transferred the family may continue with the diary).
- A diary should be started if it looks as though the patient is going to stay for a while and be sedated and ventilated.
- If a patient who was not expected to stay for a while ends up staying longer, then a summary can be done of the first few days and also from the family what had happened before coming to ICU.
- Everyone is allowed to write in the diary, but they have to sign their entry with at least their first name. Invite the relatives to contribute to the diary and read the other entries. No-one is forced to write in the diary.
- Write what you think will be important to the patient, for example if he is a football fan, he might think it is important who won the cup while he was ill. Don't be afraid to describe how serious the situation is, or else the meaning of the concept will fail.
- Take photographs of the patient when significant events happen, e.g. able to sit up for the first time for eating. Leave spaces in the diary for the photographs and write in what the photograph is of.
- The aim of the diary should be to help the patient and their family to come to terms with what happened while they were in ICU.
- When the patient leaves ICU give the diary to the relatives to let them continue the diary while the patient is still in hospital. Then when the photographs of the patient are ready invite the patient and relatives back to put the pictures in the diary (but only if the patient is mentally ready).
- Keep a record of the patient's details so that you can contact them at a later stage.
- Empty diaries should be easily available on the ICU and the diary group told if supplies are running low.

Writing a diary

The writing should be in straightforward, common language. Start the diary with a summary, which should included the reason for admission, the initial events in the ICU, and the current state of the patient's illness and the reason for doing the diary. Ask one of the relatives if they would like to summarize the course of events preceding the admission to hospital and the ICU.

Any people involved in the care of the patient, including relatives and close friends, are allowed to contribute. Any contributions should be dated. Colour pictures should be taken with a good quality camera that should not give the patient red eyes and should display the date the photograph was taken, so that the picture can be added in the appropriate place when it has been developed. The

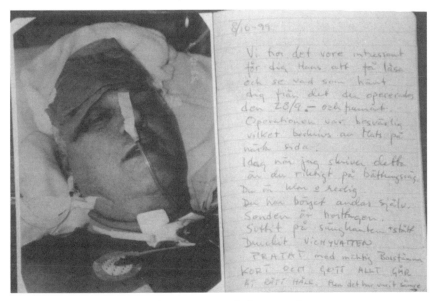

Figure 12.1 Example of a diary entry and photograph

(Translation)

*We thought it might be interesting for you Hans to read and see what has
happened since you had your operation on the 28/9 – and for the rest of the time
you will stay here.*

The operation was difficult and that is described by Mats on the next page.

Today when I'm writing this you are much better.

You are clear in your head.

You are breathing by yourself.

The gastric tube has been taken away.

You sat on the edge of your bed and also stood up.

Been drinking mineral water.

TALKED to us with a mighty baritone voice.

YOU ARE GETTING BETTER AND BETTER.

But it has been worse . . .

photographs should be realistic pictures that keep the patient's dignity and some
should be of the daily routine, with staff or relatives included.

The diary is kept by the patients' bedside until discharge from the unit.
Contributors to the diary are instructed to try to avoid too much meaningless
writing (e.g. wind and weather), but to enter everyday routines, including the
patient's reactions. The diary is brought to a close if the patient dies and this can
be either done by the family or a member of staff following discussion with the
relatives.

When the patient and relatives, or the family alone in the case of a deceased
patient, come back for a follow-up visit 2–4 weeks after discharge from the ICU,
the photographs are added to the diary with a detailed explanation of what is
happening in them. The diary can then be used as a guide to explain to the patient

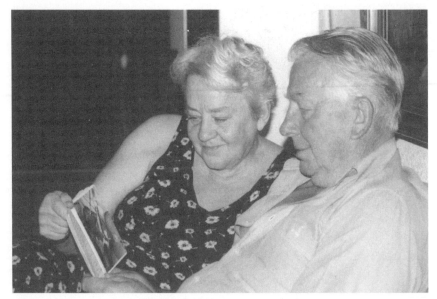

Figure 12.2 Photograph of patient and his wife reading the diary back home on the sofa

and family the course of the critical illness with the writing and photographs being explained thoroughly. The patient is given a contact telephone number so that any questions that may occur to them later can be answered, for example if someone has written that some tests have been taken the patient or their family may want to know what these are and the results.

Follow-up questionnaire

To reassure ourselves that the diaries were helping patients and their families to understand the time in ICU we decided to follow them up. The receiver of the diary was mailed a questionnaire 6 months after they were given the diary. The questions focused on how often and by whom the diary had been read. Recipients were also asked if the diary had helped them to understand the ICU stay, whether they liked having the photographs and if the writing was easy to read.

All questionnaires were answered either by the patient or their relatives. All respondents, except one teenage boy with traumatic limb amputation (who said that he would read it in the future) had shared the book with relatives and friends and claimed that it had helped them to understand their time in the ICU. They also supported the use of photographs and none had had any difficulties in understanding the writing.

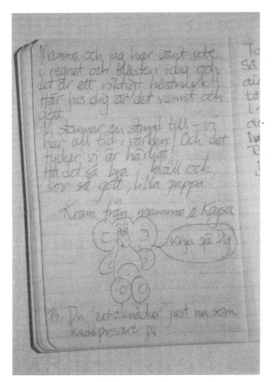

Figure 12.3 Photograph of daughter writing in her father's diary
(Translation)
*Mama and I have been out in rain and dusk today and you can feel that the
autumn is on its way!!*
But here by your side it's warm and cosy!
We will stay a little longer-we got all the time in the world!
You shall have a good evening and I hope you will sleep tight, dear papa.
Hug from mamma and Kajsa
'Hope you get better' says the elephant
PS. You are 'working extra' as a pillow tester right now. Ds

We think that our study suggests that a small investment in notebooks and
photographs and a few minutes of writing per day together with a follow-up visit
to the unit could help patients and relatives make sense of their memories or their
lack of recall.

Part

4

The greater role of aftercare

Bereavement care

Charlie Granger and Maire Shelly

Introduction

Bereavement is a universal experience. Traditionally characterized as a linear step-like path from loss to resolution, the grief process is in fact highly variable, being shaped by the individual experiences, expectations and circumstances of the bereaved (Raphael, 1984). For most people, bereavement leads eventually to an acceptance of the loss and a sense of closure. However, for a sizeable minority, possibly up to a third of the total, the process goes awry and results in a state of 'complicated grief'. Rather than progressing to eventual resolution, complicated grief is associated with continuing psychological or physical distress, and carries with it a significant risk of subsequent morbidity or mortality (Prigerson *et al.*, 1997). Identifying these vulnerable people early in the grief process may enable additional support to be offered to them, helping them to avoid the perils of complicated grief and reducing their risk of bereavement-related illness to that seen in the rest of the population (Parkes, 1980).

People whose work brings them into regular contact with death or the recently bereaved, need to be aware of the importance of handling a death in a way that assists the long-term resolution of grief, particularly for those individuals at the greatest risk of complicated grief. The development of a bereavement follow-up service may help not only the bereaved relatives but also the staff who work with the dying, who may themselves be at risk of stress-related disorders as a consequence of their work (Burke and Gerraughty, 1994).

The grief process

The grief process encompasses many stages, including shock, anger, guilt, social withdrawal and a loss of personal direction. These do not all occur in all the bereaved, neither do they occur as discrete episodes, each to be concluded before the development of the next in a predictable pathway towards resolution. Rather, bereavement has many interwoven components, which surround and assault the individual until time and the completion of the accompanying grief tasks allow the bereaved to recover their interests and appetite for life (Worden, 1982). These grief tasks require the bereaved individual to accept the reality of the death and allow them to experience the pain and grief that follow. Subsequent tasks include adjusting to the new reality of the absence of the deceased and the investment of energy and attention in new relationships and interests. Like most tasks, these are easier to accomplish with the help of others. This is broadly true both for those mourning the death of others and for patients anticipating their own death. An awareness of these stages may help when dealing with the bereaved, but what is of far more use is an appreciation of how, through sensitive and empathic care, the relatives of the dying may be encouraged to embark appropriately upon the process.

Encouraging normal grief

The grief process starts once death is predicted, rather than when it actually occurs, and involves a fundamental reappraisal of the relationship between the dying patient and their relative. Most relationships exist within a state of flux, rather than complete equilibrium – there are unfinished arguments, unspoken thoughts and unexpressed emotions. If there is no opportunity either to resolve these matters, or to accept that they are not in need of resolution before death intervenes, they may become the focus of troubling thoughts and regrets for the bereaved. As much notice as possible should therefore be given to the patient's family, and if possible to the patient as well, that there is no realistic chance of survival. The period of anticipatory grief this allows may be of irreplaceable benefit, and can be an essential component of a 'good death'. This is particularly true for children who, rather than being protected from some unpleasant truth, should be given as much time as possible to prepare for the forthcoming death of a family member (Rosenheim and Reicher, 1985). This includes encouraging parents to bring their children into the Intensive Care Unit (ICU), particularly if the patient is the other parent. If they are not allowed to see the patient, children are not only prevented from saying 'Goodbye', but may also fail to understand the finality of their relative's death or may imagine a reality far more gruesome than actually exists (Black, 1998). It is seldom appropriate, and may be directly harmful, to exclude children from the ICU, though it may seem 'right' to both the children's relatives and the ICU staff. The association between the death of a parent in childhood and subsequent mental illness should encourage us to make every possible effort to consider the needs of the children of parents dying in the ICU.

Quite apart from the need to give bad news as soon as possible, it is important that it is given by the right people, in the right way and in the right place. It is an unfortunate truth that we often fail to live up to these ideals (Cuthbertson *et al.*, 2000).

Complicated grief

Although diagnostic criteria for complicated grief have been described, the term is often used to describe any bereavement that is not proceeding 'normally'. These criteria, which include features such as a preoccupation with the deceased, refusal to accept the reality of their death or pangs of severe grief occurring over 1 year after death, allow complicated grief to be distinguished from other disorders such as depression or a post-traumatic stress disorder, which may themselves be present in 10–36% of the bereaved 2 months after death occurred (Zisook *et al.*, 1998). The consequences of complicated grief include increased risk of systemic diseases such as cancer and heart disease, as well as psychological morbidity from depression or anxiety states (Prigerson *et al.*, 1997).

The resolution of grief is influenced both by the nature of the loss suffered by the bereaved, so-called extrinsic factors (Table 13.1) and by the personal and social resources the bereaved can draw on, intrinsic factors (Table 13.2).

In many cases these factors will be predictable from knowledge either of the details of the patient's death or of the personality or circumstances of the

Table 13.1 Extrinsic factors increasing the risk of a poor outcome to bereavement

Death of a child
Loss of a parent during childhood
Sudden or early death
Violent death
Unrecovered body
'Stigmatized' death (e.g. suicide, AIDS)
Death felt to be the 'fault' of the bereaved
'Unrecognized' death – miscarriage, termination of pregnancy
Insensitively handled death

Table 13.2 Intrinsic factors increasing the risk of a poor outcome to bereavement

Low self-esteem
Previous significant psychiatric or medical disorder
Previous suicide attempt or suicidal threats
Poor social or family support
Ambivalent or dependent relationship with the deceased
Previous unresolved loss
Simultaneous significant life stresses

bereaved. However, there may also be unexpected cultural or personal factors that can only be appreciated by those who take the trouble to elicit them. In the ICU, the close relationship that often develops between the patient's family and the nursing staff may provide the ideal opportunity to unearth these factors. This relationship can also be an essential component in the development of a normal grief process, especially for individuals whose own personal or social resources are not sufficient to support them through their bereavement (Hickey and Lewandowski, 1988).

Medical staff often have a more distant relationship with a patient's relatives than do the nurses. This may be beneficial if it allows sufficient distance to make difficult medical decisions, but it should not encourage the doctor to underestimate the importance of good communication (Curtis *et al.*, 2001). Poor communication by medical staff may be a consequence of our discomfort at losing a patient or failing to cure them. It may also be the result of the low emphasis given to communication skills during medical training, although this is now being addressed by many medical schools. There are also many publications (Baile and Buckman, 1998) that aim to ease this problem and which may help to improve the reputation of the profession for communicating bad news, though to benefit from these resources we have first to concede that our communication skills can be improved (Levy, 2001).

Talking to relatives

The way in which families are informed about a relative's poor prognosis may be something they never forget. Giving families this news, just as for any other family conference, should be approached with as much care as any other ICU procedure and, in the correct circumstances, may provide an equally valuable opportunity for teaching junior staff (Curtis *et al.*, 2001). Talking to the family before the patient's death is the first step in post-bereavement care and can ease post-bereavement care considerably.

Where to give bad news

Sensitive discussions with families should be held in a room designed for the purpose (Intensive Care Society, 1998). The room should be welcoming, comfortably furnished and large enough for a reasonably sized family. The family should be encouraged to use the room for as long as they need it once the bad news has been given.

How to give bad news

In the popular imagination the ICU is associated with death. Most relatives will, therefore, have at least a subconscious expectation that things may go badly and, in many cases, the family will be all too aware that there is no realistic chance of recovery. Some families have previous experience of an ICU that will colour their preconceptions. It is important to remember that the delivery of the message includes both the words and the body language employed.

The family conference should include the immediate family members, unless particular circumstances dictate otherwise. It is also helpful to have another member of staff present, usually this will be the patient's nurse, whose role at the conference extends beyond just comforting the family and acting as a witness to what has been said. The nurse may also be able to prompt the family to ask questions they have already asked her which, quite apart from its service to the family, may also improve her professional satisfaction with the end-of-life care she is able to deliver (Asch *et al.*, 1997; Curtis *et al.*, 2001).

At the start of the conversation with the family it is important to find out what they understand of the patient's condition. In many cases this will reveal that all that is necessary is to confirm their fears and the language they use will help the doctor pitch his explanation at the appropriate level. Once it is clear what information needs to be given, it is important to try to give the facts clearly and in small comprehensible chunks. It may be helpful to start with a warning, such as 'I'm afraid I've got some bad news for you'. This will warn the family of the significance of the impending news and give them a moment to prepare for what is to come. If there is a lot to say, understanding should be checked at regular intervals, and the pace of delivery adjusted to the family's pace of reception. Essential facts should be repeated for emphasis. It is crucial that bad news is given honestly. Families particularly need to trust the doctors caring for critically ill relatives so the temptation of encouraging either false hope, or prognostic certainty in the presence of doubt, should be resisted. Unfortunately, it is apparent that, in spite of our best efforts, relatives do not always hear what we think we have told them (Levy, 2001), so at the end of the family conference it is wise to offer a synopsis of what has been said, to stress the most important points and to repeat whatever management plan has been agreed.

Families may not react to bad news as expected: anger, overwhelming distress or an apparent absence of grief may be particularly difficult to deal with. In the face of anger personal offence should not be taken. Rather, sensitive non-judgemental handling will usually be effective. Equally, it is not always appropriate for the doctor to distance themselves from the family's distress: emotional honesty may be a support to the family, so it may be more appropriate to show that you share some part of the family's distress rather than to try to hide it behind a shield of professional detachment (Levy, 2001). Such a level of involvement by the doctor may come at a personal price, and doctors should be encouraged to develop coping strategies to deal with the undoubted stresses involved (Ptacek *et al.*, 1999). The process of clinical supervision (see Chapter 15) may be invaluable in dealing with these stresses.

Who should give bad news

Bad news should usually be delivered by the most senior intensive care doctor involved in the patient's care and should be consistent (Johnson *et al.*, 1998).

Follow-up and support

Any bereavement follow-up programme should be designed to address a number of issues:

- The delivery of appropriate support and information to the bereaved to help to normalize the bereavement process.
- Gathering information on the family's experiences of end-of-life care and providing feedback to the staff.
- Seeking suggestions about how end-of-life care may be improved.
- Providing an avenue for intensive care staff to obtain support when required.

The delivery of support

The experience of grief is unique to the grieving individual. There should, therefore, be a variety in the range of support services available to help each individual in their grief. The simplest and least threatening way to offer support to the bereaved is to send a 'Condolences' card, or for a member of staff known to the family to phone them to offer support (Burke and Gerraughty, 1994; Campbell and Thill, 2000). At this time, if the family have any questions relating to the patient's hospital stay, they can be offered the opportunity to meet the nursing or medical staff who were involved in the patient's care, as well as given details about other sources of information or support (Intensive Care Society, 1998; Kojlak et al., 1998; Campbell and Thill, 2000). The nature of the support offered can vary from simply answering questions the family did not feel able to ask at the time, to reviewing the course of events leading to death, or hospital or community-based bereavement counselling from trained staff. The support offered should be sufficient to encourage a normal bereavement process for each individual.

A successful bereavement programme needs to be able to provide whatever resources are required, and there is good evidence that these forms of support are welcomed by the bereaved, especially after particularly traumatic events such as the death of a child. Unfortunately, for some people, accepting the offer of bereavement support carries with it the stigma of not being able to cope, which may reduce the take-up of a valuable and effective service. Thereafter, further contact may be made with the bereaved at varying intervals, usually ending with a card on the first anniversary of the death (Campbell and Thill, 2000). Some staff may find the idea of a bereavement support programme threatening, so care should be taken to ensure that staff are not obliged to take part if they feel uncomfortable with it, but should be allowed time to see its value to others and join in as they feel ready (Burke and Gerraughty, 1994).

Gathering information and providing feedback

Most studies of bereaved relatives have demonstrated consistent strengths and weaknesses in the provision of end-of-life care. These demonstrate that good communication skills among critical care staff, continuity of care and compassion are the most highly valued assets (Cuthbertson *et al.*, 2000; Curtis *et al.*, 2001). Not surprisingly, poor communication is identified as the most significant problem (Cuthbertson *et al.*, 2000; Levy, 2001). For any particular ICU, the balance between these strengths and weaknesses can only be discovered by asking patients' families, and this can most easily and consistently be done during bereavement follow-up. This information should be passed back to the critical care staff to give them the opportunity to try to develop their weaknesses and reinforce their strengths (Cuthbertson *et al.*, 2000). Nursing the dying can be highly rewarding if end-of-life care is delivered in the way in which the patient, their family and the staff feel appropriate, although it is apparent that neither the family nor the staff will necessarily be correct in their assumptions about what the patient really wants. Nursing the dying can also be a source of great frustration if the care delivered appears to be incompatible with the patient's wishes (Asch *et al.*, 1997). In some cases this frustration can even lead to staff complying with requests for euthanasia, in spite of professional or legal prohibitions against it (Asch and DeKay, 1997).

Learning from the family

Irrespective of the best endeavours by the ICU staff, patients and their families may not receive the end-of-life care they desire. This may result from discussions about end-of-life care being held too late to influence care, possibly because both the physician and the family are waiting for the other to introduce the subject (Larson and Tobin, 2000). In other units the lay-out of the unit may make compassionate end-of-life care difficult (Levy, 2001), or staff may unwittingly not give relatives permission to be physically close to the patient as they are dying (Pierce, 1999). Staff involved in running bereavement follow-up programmes should make use of the opportunity it presents to ask families for their suggestions about improving the experience of dying in their ICU.

Supporting staff

There is no doubt that caring for the dying can be stressful for staff (Asch and DeKay, 1997; Johnson *et al.*, 1998), especially if they feel untrained for the responsibility it places on them. These stresses may place staff at risk of emotional fatigue and 'burnout', which may be associated with excessive alcohol use and increased staff turnover. It may also explain why staff who agree on the factors that should lead to a decision to withdraw care from a patient in practice vary widely when they make the decision to do so (Cook *et al.*, 1995). A bereavement support programme can significantly reduce the stress experienced by staff caring for the dying, both by providing positive feedback to them from the patients' families and by allowing them to shape the way end-of-life care is delivered on their unit (Hodges and Graham, 1988; Johnson *et al.*, 1993; Burke and Gerraughty, 1994).

Conclusion

Bereavement may be associated with significant long-term morbidity. Knowledge of the factors that may lead to this outcome permits timely referral to suitable support services. Early provision of appropriate support reduces the risk of bereavement-related illness and should be the responsibility of all those dealing regularly with the terminally ill. Sensitive handling of grieving relatives is an essential step towards establishing a good bereavement. The benefits of a bereavement follow-up service for both staff and bereaved families are indisputable (Raphael, 1977; Johnson *et al.*, 1993) and the development of a bereavement service should be considered by all with an interest in intensive care.

References

Asch DA, DeKay ML Euthanasia among US critical care nurses. Practices, attitudes and social and professional correlates. *Medical Care* 1997; **35**, 890–900.

Asch DA, Shea JA, Jedrziewski MK, Bosk CL The limits of suffering: critical care nurses' views of hospital care at the end of life. *Social Science and Medicine* 1997; **45**, 1661–8.

Baile W, Buckman R *The Pocket Guide to Communication Skills in Clinical Practice including Breaking Bad News*. Medical Audio-Visual Communications Inc. email:dwc-@mavc.com, 1998.

Black D Bereavement in childhood. *British Medical Journal* 1998; **316**, 931–3.

Burke C, Gerraughty SM An oncology unit's initiation of a bereavement support program. *Oncological Nursing Forum* 1994; **21**, 1675–80.

Campbell ML, Thill M Bereavement follow-up to families after death in the intensive care unit. *Critical Care Medicine* 2000; **28**, 1252–3.

Cook DJ, Guyatt GH, Jaeschke R *et al.* Determinants in Canadian health care workers of the decision to withdraw life support from the critically ill. Canadian Critical Care Trials Group. *Journal of the American Medical Association* 1995; **273**, 703–8.

Curtis JR, Patrick DL, Shannon SE *et al.* The family conference as a focus to improve communication about end-of-life care in the intensive care unit: opportunities for improvement. *Critical Care Medicine* 2001; **29**(Suppl.), N26–33.

Cuthbertson SJ, Margetts MA, Streat SJ Bereavement follow-up after critical illness. *Critical Care Medicine* 2000; **28**, 1196–201.

Hickey M, Lewandowski L Critical care nurses' role with families: a descriptive study. *Heart and Lung* 1988: **17**, 670–6.

Hodge DS, Graham PL A hospital-based neonatal intensive care unit bereavement program: an evaluation of its effectiveness. *Journal of Perinatology* 1988; **8**, 247–52.

Intensive Care Society. *Guidelines for Bereavement Care in Intensive Care Units.* The Intensive Care Society, London: 1998.

Johnson D, Wilson M, Cavanaugh B *et al.* Measuring the ability to meet family needs in an intensive care unit. *Critical Care Medicine* 1998; **26**, 266–71.

Johnson LC, Rincon B, Gober C, Rexin D The development of a comprehensive bereavement program to assist families experiencing pediatric loss. *Journal of Pediatric Nursing* 1993; **8**, 142–6.

Kojlak K, Keenan SP, Plotkin D *et al.* Determining the potential need for a bereavement follow-up program: how well are family and health care workers' needs currently being met? *Journal of the Canadian Association of Critical Care News* 1998; **9**, 12–16.

Larson DG, Tobin DR End-of-life conversations: evolving practice and theory. *Journal of the American Medical Association* 2000; **284**, 1573–8.

Levy MM End-of-life care in the intensive care unit: Can we do better? *Critical Care Medicine* 2001; **29**(Suppl.), N56–N61.

Parkes CM Bereavement counselling: Does it work? *British Medical Journal* 1980; **281**, 3–6.

Pierce SF Improving end-of-life care: gathering suggestions from family members. *Nursing Forum* 1999; **34**, 5–14.

Prigerson HG, Bierhals AJ, Kasl SV *et al.* Traumatic grief as a risk factor for mental and physical morbidity. *American Journal of Psychiatry* 1997; **154**, 616–23.

Ptacek JT, Fries EA, Eberhardt TL Breaking bad news to patients: physicians perceptions of the process. *Supportive Care in Cancer* 1999; **7**, 113–20.

Raphael B Preventive intervention with the recently bereaved. *Archives of General Psychiatry* 1977; **34**, 1450–4.

Raphael B *The Anatomy of Bereavement.* Hutchinson, London: 1984.

Rosenheim E, Reicher R Informing children about a parent's terminal illness. *Journal of Child Psychology and Psychiatry* 1985; **26**, 995–8.

Worden JW *Grief Counselling and Grief Therapy. A Handbook for the Mental Health Practitioner.* Springer Publishing, New York: 1982.

Zisook S, Chentsova-Dutton Y, Shuchter SR Post-traumatic stress disorder following bereavement. *Annals of Clinical Psychology* 1998; **10**, 157–63.

Classification and measurement problems of outcomes after intensive care

Saxon Ridley and Duncan Young

Introduction

Severely ill patients entering intensive care units receive treatment for their primary condition as well as general supportive measures to maintain homeostasis while the specific therapy takes effect. In the past intensive care has tended to be regarded as a 'black box'; patients enter an intensive care unit, receive a package of care and are discharged to the ward or die. It has been difficult to unravel and identify the individual processes and procedures that make up intensive care and the effects of intensive care on mortality or morbidity persisting after discharge from the intensive care unit have largely been ignored. However, increasing pressure on healthcare resources coupled with better informed patients and their relatives necessitates a far more sophisticated approach. As part of this approach it is necessary to examine carefully a whole range of outcomes from intensive care, not simply intensive care unit mortality, so that the effectiveness and efficiency of the individual components of intensive care can be examined.

Measuring outcome following intensive care is not easy. Intensive care is a relatively modern development in medicine, and has a short history of outcome studies. There is a wide variety of outcome measures devised by other disciplines and applied to many patient groups, but clearly not all of these are useful to physicians involved in intensive care or meaningful to their patients. Randomized controlled trials, which are a major stimulus to the development of outcome measures, have been only slowly accepted in intensive care because of the severe illness of the patients and the natural tendency to use all therapeutic options in an attempt to save lives. Despite these limitations, enough is now known about some outcome measures in intensive care for them to be usefully applied so that variations between outcomes can be explored and some of the possible controlling influences identified.

This chapter briefly outlines one possible classification of outcomes following intensive care, illustrates this classification with examples and highlights some of the problems with the measurement of outcome. The reader is directed to a sister publication 'Outcome measures in intensive care' (Ridley and Young, 2002).

Classification of outcomes after intensive care

Outcomes from intensive care can be viewed from at least three perspectives; that of the patients, the clinical staff and the managers of the healthcare system (Figure 14.1). Different measures will be required to investigate the areas of interest to each of the three groups.

Patients and relatives

The patient's perspective, as the consumer and end user of the healthcare system, is of prime importance. Their interest focuses on survival, quality of life and functional ability once they have recovered from critical illness.

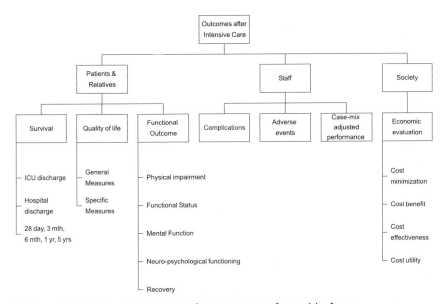

Figure 14.1 A classification tree for outcomes after critical care

1 Survival

Survival is a key outcome measure. It is clearly of great importance to the patients and their relatives but also to the attendant staff as it provides some crude idea of the effectiveness of modern medical management and allows the assessment of medical advances. Survival following critical illness has been measured at ICU discharge, hospital discharge and at random calendar periods (e.g. 28 days, 6 months, 1 and 5 years) following admission to ICU.

Survival to ICU discharge is clearly of major interest to patients and relatives. The majority of patients who die in spite of receiving intensive care do so in the intensive care unit. When relatives enquire about a patient's chances of dying they usually expect information on the chance of dying on the intensive care unit rather than at some later point in their hospital stay or after discharge. Deaths within the intensive care unit are determined by at least two broad categories of factors. The first category relates to the patient and the second to the organization applied to the process of intensive care delivery. The patient factors are the same as those that determine survival to hospital discharge, namely the influences of advancing age, presence of significant co-morbidities (such as diabetes, cancer, immunosuppression and chronic organ dysfunction), level of physiological derangement, the underlying cause of the critical illness and whether the patient was admitted as an emergency. To compare survival rates at intensive care discharge over time or between units these variations in the patient population (i.e. the case-mix) have to be corrected for. There is a variety of severity scoring systems that allow correction for case-mix when examining intensive care unit, as opposed to hospital, mortality. Examples are the PRISM (paediatric risk of mortality) score (Pollack *et al.*, 1988) in children and the SOFA (sequential organ failure assessment) score (Vincent *et al.*, 1996) in adults.

Organizational factors that influence hospital mortality include the timing of delivery of intensive care, the internal organization of the intensive care unit in terms of whether the unit is 'open' (i.e. clinical management retained by referring doctor) or 'closed' (where ICU management is delivered by an intensive care specialist) (Carson *et al.*, 1996) and if there is an efficient and effective communication system between all types of staff (Knaus *et al.*, 1986). However, intensive care unit mortality is rarely used by researchers because it is heavily influenced by the site where patients are cared for after intensive care has been deemed futile. In addition, if it were discussed with them in detail, patients would want to know their chance of leaving the hospital alive, rather than leaving the intensive care unit alive only to die on the ward.

Hospital mortality is an extremely frequently quoted outcome measure. While a patient is receiving intensive care, the question mainly asked by their relatives is whether the patient is going to survive. Once the patient has been discharged to the general ward, the question changes to what quality of life the patient is likely to enjoy. This emphasizes an important but subtle change in the patient's and relative's perception of outcome. The relatives may be understandably disappointed if the patient dies in hospital having survived the rigours of intensive care. Alas, post-intensive care but within hospital mortality can be extremely high. In Europe, the post-intensive care hospital mortality varies between 23 and 31% of all admissions (Moreno and Agthe, 1999). From the intensive care staff's perspective, hospital mortality may not be viewed as a particularly useful outcome measure as it reflects the performance of the whole hospital episode and hence the entire institution's performance of which the intensive care unit may only be one part. By and large intensive care staff do not play a significant role in the management of patients once they have returned to the general ward. As a result, hospital mortality measures institutional rather than intensive care performance, including the effects of care before and after the stay in intensive care. Despite this significant limitation, hospital mortality is the predicted outcome for several severity of illness scores and performance indicators used by regulatory agencies. Examples of these are the various versions of the Acute Physiology and Chronic Health Evaluation (APACHE) scores (Knaus et al., 1991), the Mortality Prediction Models (MPM) (Lemeshow et al., 1993) and the Simplified Acute Physiology Scoring (SAPS) system (Le Gall et al., 1993).

The patients and their relatives may regard a return to an independent existence in the community as a therapeutic success. They will be interested in the expected duration of long-term survival. Unfortunately, the long-term survival of critically ill patients in the UK has been shown to be less favourable than that of an age- and sex-matched population (Ridley and Plenderleith, 1994). This may relate to the underlying diagnosis, the effects of severe physiological disturbance or probably both. At the moment, the length of time it takes for the survival curve of a group of critically ill patients to match that of an age- and sex-matched normal population is unknown. Results from European studies suggest that this may take place in a relatively short period of time varying between 6 months and a year. On the other hand, data from the UK, where intensive care beds are less numerous and the patients in them generally more ill, suggest that it takes several years (in excess of three) for the critically ill survivors to have the same mortality rate as the normal population (Lam and Ridley, 1999).

In some groups of patients, long-term survival following critical illness is poor. These groups include medical (as opposed to surgical) patients, the very elderly (patients aged over 85 years), patients with incurable cancer and patients admitted with significant co-morbid disease such as diabetes, steroid therapy and more than two organ failures. Using general severity of illness scores, it is possible to predict the chances of hospital survival; unfortunately, not enough is known about the influences on long-term survival for accurate estimates of future life expectancy to be given. In the UK, this area of important research is largely hindered by the difficulty in following patients once they return to the community. Differences in the case-mix of critically ill patients between countries may mean that results from one country cannot be applied to another.

2 Quality of life

Quality of life is one of the most important non-mortality outcome measures after critical illness. Quality of life may be defined as a concept encompassing a broad range of physical and psychological characteristics and limitations that describe an individual's ability to function in their environment and derive satisfaction from so doing. Health related quality of life describes the level of well-being of the individual's life as affected by accident, injury, disease and treatments.

Quality of life is a key outcome measure as it is one of the main attributes relating to the enjoyment of life in general. Quality of life is difficult to quantify as it is influenced by a large number of factors including many outside the control of the healthcare system and it varies when measured over time. Changes in quality of life may not necessarily be related to simple biological variables, such as blood pressure, and at the moment our understanding of the control of the physiological and psychological aspects of quality of life is extremely limited.

Notwithstanding the difficulties involved in measurement of quality of life, attempts to measure it have been made in many spheres of medicine outside intensive care. Quality of life in patients with chronic conditions such as hypertension, diabetes, rheumatoid arthritis and parkinsonism have been frequently studied. Because of the acute nature of critical illness and its relatively transient effects (compared with life-long diseases such as diabetes), the measurement of quality of life following critical illness is difficult because of the relatively rapid changes over time.

Quality of life measures may be divided into disease-specific or general measures. Specific measures should be used for the disease process, such as hypertension or diabetes, for which they were specifically designed. In the intensive care setting, quality of life has been most frequently measured using general tools such as the Sickness Impact Profile (Bergner *et al.*, 1981), Nottingham Health Profile (Hunt *et al.*, 1985) and the Short Form 36 (Ware *et al.*, 1993). The results from studies are not comprehensive. Despite their age, quality of life in elderly patients seems to be related more to the severity of illness and admitting diagnosis rather than age itself. In young trauma victims, however, quality of life can be adversely affected after their accident or injury. There are indications that patients who are most severely ill and those who stay longest in intensive care either have long-lasting changes in quality of life or make the slowest recovery of quality of life.

Part of the problem relating to quality of life measurement concerns the actual process and timing of measurement. For example, Gill and Feinstein (1994) randomly selected 75 articles reporting quality of life after critical illness and found that 136 out of 159 of the measures used had been used only once. Such diversity of measures used only once makes comparisons between studies difficult. When assessing intensive care, investigators frequently fail to report the psychometric properties (validity and reliability) of the instrument they use and rarely report the steps they have taken to ensure adequacy of the sample size. Most of the outcome measures that have been used in intensive care research, the frequency with which they have been used and their psychometric properties are more fully presented in a systematic review undertaken by the Intensive Care National Audit and Research Centre (ICNARC) (Hayes *et al.*, 2000); readers are urged to use this as a reference work on outcome measures. Investigators should be encouraged to select the tools that are specifically designed for the area of outcome in which they are interested (e.g. physical impairment, functional status, mental or neuropsychological function, recovery or quality of life).

We do not know enough about the interaction of the primary pathology and the undesirable complications of intensive care management. For example, victims of serious road traffic accidents may develop post-traumatic stress disorder, but intensive care unit treatment itself can lead to psychosis, anxiety and depression. How much of the patient's psychological change is due to their presenting injury or illness rather than the effects of their management is simply unknown. Whatever the relationship, psychological consequences of the accident or treatment are likely to have serious and adverse effects on the patient's quality of life.

As with survival, alterations in quality of life are the result of the whole hospital episode, and intensive care management is only a part of this process. Quality of life (and functional outcome), like long-term survival, is dependent upon the effectiveness of the whole healthcare system, including support received in the convalescent period while in the community. Without carefully controlling the effects of support after intensive care, it may be unwise to ascribe changes in long-term outcome measures to intensive care unit management alone.

3 Functional outcome

Functional outcome describes physical or mental capability and capacity. Functional outcome and quality of life are often used interchangeably but this is incorrect because functional outcome does not include any measure of satisfaction or well-being. Functional outcome is not dependent upon personal perceptions and so may be both easier to measure and capable of being objectively measured by a researcher. The patients' perception and satisfaction with life may vary independently of functional outcome. The recovery of functional outcome over time may not parallel the recovery of quality of life. For example, after life-threatening illness, the patients may enjoy a good quality of life, being thankful for being alive or may have a poorer quality of life being resentful of the long-term physical effects of the injuries or disease.

Functional outcome can be divided into five areas:

a Physical impairment and disability

Physical impairment and disability will be common after severe trauma but its measurement may not be appropriate for other causes of critical illness. Because ventilation is a key therapeutic modality in intensive care, measures of physical impairment have concentrated on the respiratory system and have included measures of pulmonary function, such as spirometry and diffusing capacity, as well as measures of long-standing upper airway damage using endoscopy and radiological examination. Alas these outcome measures have rather limited application in outcome analysis except for those patients admitted with acute lung injury and other causes of severe respiratory impairment, or those who have had a surgical airway created during their stay. Most patients who recover from the acute respiratory distress syndrome develop a restrictive defect upon recovery; fortunately this generally does not impair patients unless they undertake strenuous physical activity.

b Functional status

Functional status measures may be broadly classified as disease-specific or general measures. The New York Heart Association (NYHA) classification has been used in critically ill patients, but this tool was originally designed for patients suffering with congestive cardiac failure (Criteria Committee of the New York Association, 1964). The classification grades physical activities. General measures of functional status include the ability to perform the activities of daily living (bathing, dressing, going to the toilet, moving, continence and feeding) and these have been modified into the instrumental activities of daily living (using the telephone, shopping, using transport, cooking, housekeeping, taking medicine and handling finances). Unfortunately, most outcome measures examining functional status were developed for use in other fields. For example, Katz's activities of daily living (ADL) were originally developed from results obtained from elderly patients with fractured neck of femur (Katz et al., 1970). The application of the activities of daily living as a primary outcome measure to intensive care survivors may therefore be flawed.

Even so, the activities of daily living have been used in a number of studies examining patients' functional outcomes following critical illness. In elderly patients, functional outcome appears to return to pre-morbid levels after 6 months to a year (Chelluri et al., 1993) and there was no difference in recovery of function status between those over and under 65 years of age (Rockwood et al., 1993). In a general adult ICU population of 1746 patients, the SUPPORT study reported a tripling in incidence (to 34%) of severe functional limitations at 2 months; unfortunately this particular study did not follow the patients for longer so it is not known how many improved or deteriorated further (Wu et al., 1995). Following neurosurgical intensive care, recovery of functional status at a mean follow-up time of 2.2 years (range 1–3 years) as measured by activities of daily living was poor. Only 23% of 122 survivors scored above the threshold value for moderate to minimal disability (Cho and Wang, 1997).

c Mental function

As with functional status, mental function outcome measures may be divided into generic measures and disease-specific measures. An example of a generic measure is the Profile of Mood State (POMS) (McNair et al., 1992). This scale was developed to assess mood in psychiatric outpatients. The scale assesses mood by ranking 65 adjectives on a five-point scale. The Hospital Anxiety and Depression Scale (HADS) was developed in non-psychiatric patients to measure mood disorders and depression; it contains 14 items asking about depression and anxiety (Zigmond and Snaith, 1983). Mood changes are some of the commonest sequelae of critical illness and intensive care support.

Disease-specific mental function tests include the Impact of Events Scale (IES) and this assesses psychological distress following trauma (Horowitz *et al.*, 1979). The IES has been used outside intensive care for measuring post-traumatic stress in individuals following disasters such as oil-rig sinking and fires. The IES consists of 15 symptom-items that respondents rate according to the frequency of occurrence in the last 7 days, on a scaled mark 0 (*Not at all*), 1 (*Fairly*), 3 (*Sometimes*) and 5 (*Often*). It has two sub-scales, the first pertains to re-experiencing the trauma (e.g. nightmares) and contains seven items, while the second sub-scale refers to avoiding situations and thoughts that are associated with the trauma (eight items). Scores on the IES sub-scales for intrusions and avoidance have been stratified as <9 mild or absent symptoms, 9–19 medium level of symptoms and over 20 high levels of symptoms (maximum possible score 75). Scores above 30 on the IES indicate severe psychological trauma symptoms and individuals scoring in this range are likely to meet diagnostic criteria for post-traumatic stress disorder. Scores on the IES are skewed; individuals who are not psychologically traumatized score close to zero while those who have suffered a wide range of traumatic experiences achieved higher scores. Patients recovering from severe non-central nervous system traumatic injury have a mean score of 30.6 at 3 months after injury.

d Neuropsychological function

This measures cognitive function and examples include Trailmaking Tests A and B, Wisconsin Card Sorting Test and Benton's test for visual retention. The tests are generally used as part of a battery of tests assessing neuropsychological function in association with central nervous system disorders. The tests are complex and usually require face-to-face interviews. They measure attention, perception, cognitive flexibility, information processing and visual memory. These tests have been used for patients with head injury, but are probably rather limited for the general intensive care patient because of their complex application and primary role in assessing brain dysfunction.

e Measures of recovery

The extent of recovery may be measured in a multi-item scale such as the Glasgow Outcome Scale which has four grades of recovery (good, moderate disability, severe disability and vegetative state) (Jennett and Bond, 1975). The scale was originally intended to assess recovery 6 months after head injury. However, it was expanded and used to show that mental handicap (usually personality changes) contributed more significantly to overall social disability than did neurological (i.e. physical) deficits. Simple single item scales such as returning to work or independent living have been used, but their simplicity limits their usefulness as there are many grades of employment and varying levels of support available to maintain independence.

The measurement of functional outcome following intensive care is subject to the same problems as measurement of quality of life. The validity and reliability of the tools used following critical illness have not been demonstrated adequately. Similarly the responsiveness and recovery of functional outcome following critical illness is unknown. Whether or not the recovery of functional outcome parallels that of quality of life is simply unknown. Function outcome, however, is an extremely important outcome measure from the patient's perspective.

Staff's perspective

The intensive care unit staff are interested in outcome measures that relate to their professional performance. Measuring outcome and performance is difficult because the capabilities and capacity of any intensive care unit will be influenced by the case-mix of patients. However, performance can be measured in at least two ways. The professional standards of care attained by the staff may be measured in terms of the incidence of complications or accidents arising in intensive care. Should these adverse events lead to morbidity then clearly these outcome measures are also of interest to the patients and their relatives as well. The overall performance of intensive care can be measured using case-mix adjusted severity of illness scores to produce comparisons of the observed to expected mortality (otherwise known as the standardized mortality ratio). National programmes such as ICNARC's case-mix programme provide valuable information regarding the comparative performance of individual units.

1 Complications

Adverse events and complications may reflect the standard of care delivered on the intensive care unit and so will be of interest to staff. Cross-infection rates may reflect professional standards of practice and, in Europe, higher rates of nosocomial infection have been linked to higher intensive care unit mortality rates. Adverse events and complications may be pathology dependent (for example, amputation of peripheries because of ischaemia or extensive bowel resection leading to prolonged dependence on total parenteral nutrition) or they may be treatment dependent. Treatment dependent complications can be divided into general complications such as weight loss, critical illness neuropathy and joint stiffness or specific treatment related complications such as tracheal stenosis following tracheostomy.

Unfortunately, complications occur commonly on intensive care units. Giraud recorded 316 iatrogenic complications in 124 out of 400 admissions (31%) in two centres in France (Giraud et al., 1993). The commonest complications involved ventilator procedures or therapeutic errors. This distribution of complications was confirmed by the Australian Incident Monitoring Study (AIMS) (Beckmann et al., 1996) which analysed 610 complications involving drugs (28%), procedures (23%), patient environment (21%), airway (20%) and ICU management (9%). Some complications may be categorized as both treatment and pathology dependent.

2 Case-mix adjusted performance

Using any of the APACHE scoring systems, the MPM models or the SAPS scoring system, it is possible to calculate a predicted risk of hospital death for each patient admitted to intensive care. This can be compared with the actual mortality to produce a standardized mortality ratio. Despite the reservations concerning the use of a single crude outcome measure like mortality and the dependence of such mortality estimates on correctly recorded physiological data, comparisons of standardized mortality ratios provide some useful information. For example, Figure 14.2 shows the distribution of the standardized mortality ratios of ICUs contributing to ICNARC Case-Mix Programme calculated using the APACHE II system calibrated for UK patients in the late 1980s.

This diagram suggests that most units in the UK have a higher than expected mortality across the entire range of mortality predictions. Whether this reflects a declining intensive care unit performance, a change in the calibration of the APACHE II system over time, or a change in case-mix that renders the previous calibration unreliable, is debated. In addition, because of the statistical uncertainty in the estimates of standardized mortality ratios, very few ICUs have a standardized mortality ratio significantly different from 1 on statistical testing. However, what cannot be denied is that such figures produce considerable interest and may act as a stimulus to attain the highest possible professional standards.

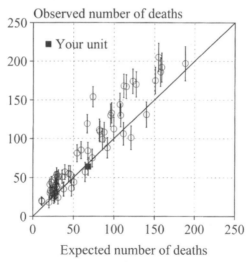

Figure 14.2 A scatter diagram of the standardized mortality ratios (i.e. the observed number of deaths against the expected number of deaths) for the critical care units participating in the case-mix programme of the Intensive Care National Audit and Research Centre. The highlighted unit ('Your unit') is the Critical Care Complex at the Norfolk and Norwich Acute NHS Trust. (Diagram reproduced from the Intensive Care National Audit and Research Centre's Case Mix Programme Data Analysis Report to the Norfolk and Norwich Acute NHS Trust for period 01/06/99 to 28/11/99.)

Predicting a patient's death is an inexact science and sometimes a balance needs to be struck between exploring every avenue of organ support in an attempt to save the patient's life against exposing the patient to intrusive, undignified, prolonged and ultimately futile intervention. The identification of futility is difficult; at present no perfect system exists. However, organ failure scores, which sequentially monitor organ dysfunction, can generate a useful and objective way of demonstrating increasing physiological derangement. Demonstrating a failure of intensive care supportive measures to reverse the physiological decline might be one factor taken into account when reaching decisions concerning altering the aims of intensive care. Sequential organ scoring has been shown to be an effective method of identifying adverse physiological trends and a means of maintaining standards of care. Sequential SOFA, APACHE II and APACHE III scores have been used in this way.

Society's perspective

Health managers, economists and politicians are not necessarily interested in an individual's prognosis or clinical problems. Their task involves distributive justice to maximize the good for the whole of society. They are required to make rational decisions about healthcare resourcing based on accurate and reliable data. They must resolve conflicts concerning areas of healthcare, not only within hospital but also in trying to establish the appropriate balance between primary and secondary healthcare.

Such decision making should be based upon rigorous economic evaluation using techniques of cost-minimization, cost-effectiveness, cost-benefit and cost-utility analyses. The selection of the appropriate technique once again depends upon the perspective chosen. For example, Trust managers may focus on cost-minimization studies in an attempt to reduce hospital expenditure. Policy makers in the Department of Health will be more interested in cost-effectiveness or cost-utility measures in order to balance decisions about healthcare investment. The other arm of such evaluation is, of course, the accurate measurement of cost. Intensive care is very expensive, but surprisingly cost is infrequently measured. Indeed, in a review of 20 years of published reports commenting on intensive care unit costs, Gyldmark (1995) found only 20 studies reporting a cost methodology in sufficient detail to allow it to be repeated. Even then, there were omissions or methodological problems or biases in at least half of these studies. These problems partly arise because intensive care delivery is dependent upon, and contributed to, by many other hospital departments. Costing methods are being developed and hopefully a validated, simple, but reasonably accurate method will evolve.

The data required for such outcome measures will probably be of little interest to the critically ill individual presenting to an intensive care unit. However, for the professionals involved in intensive care, one of the pressing tasks must be to produce accurate and reliable information to allow rational decision making.

These data are important because we have a duty to ensure that we are not profligate with hospital resources.

The division of resources involves measurement of cost and benefit and then comparison with other competing healthcare programmes. Such comparisons require reduction of outcome into common comparable units of outcome. These units of outcome may be obvious for certain forms of treatment. For example, the comparison between two antihypertensive drugs may result in a mean reduction of 20 mmHg (for the purposes of argument) in one group compared to another. When this reduction is related to the difference in costs between the two antihypertensive drugs, then the units of outcome may be expressed as a change of mmHg per £ spent (or saved) depending upon the drug. Unfortunately, for intensive care, the outcome comparison is once again limited by the lack of a control group. The median survival times may be quoted and may be adjusted by combination with a measure of quality of life to produce a theoretical outcome unit such as a 'Quality Adjusted Life Year' (QALY). In this way QALYs or median survival times after intensive care can be compared to other healthcare programmes.

Summary

Outcomes measures used for intensive care are almost as varied as the patients we treat. They may vary from purely patient based and orientated to outcomes of interest to healthcare providers. Because of outside influences and the general supportive nature of intensive care, the outcome chosen for measurement of benefit or effectiveness requires careful selection. Our problem in intensive care is not that intensive care and high-dependency units are not delivering high quality supportive care, but rather that we have not defined the correct goals and outcome measurements to demonstrate their worth.

References

Beckmann U, West LF, Groombridge GJ et al. The Australian incident monitoring study in intensive care: AIMS-ICU. The development and evaluation of an incident reporting system in intensive care. Anaesthesia and Intensive Care 1996; **24**, 314–19.

Bergner M, Bobbitt RA, Carter WB, Gilson BS The Sickness Impact Profile: development and final revision of a health status measure. Medical Care 1981; **19**, 787–805.

Carson SS, Stocking C, Podsadecki T et al. Effects of organizational change in the medical intensive care unit of a teaching hospital: a comparison of 'open' and 'closed' formats. Journal of the American Medical Association 1996; **276**, 322–8.

Chelluri L, Pinsky MR, Donahoe MP, Grenvik A Long-term outcome of critically ill elderly patients requiring intensive care. Journal of the American Medical Association 1993; **269**, 3119–23.

Cho D-Y, Wang Y-C Comparison of the APACHE III, APACHE II, and Glasgow Coma Scale in acute head injury for prediction of mortality and functional outcome. Intensive Care Medicine 1997; **23**, 77–84.

Criteria Committee of the New York Heart Association Nomenclature and Criteria for Diagnosis of Disease of the Heart and Blood Vessels. Little Brown, Boston: 1964.

Gill TM, Feinstein AR A critical appraisal of the quality of quality-of-life measurements. *Journal of the American Medical Association* 1994; **272**, 619–26.

Giraud T, Dhainaut JF, Vaxelaire JF *et al.* Iatrogenic complications in adult intensive care units: a prospective two-center study. *Critical Care Medicine* 1993; **21**, 40–51.

Gyldmark M A review of cost studies of intensive care units: problems with the cost concept. *Critical Care Medicine* 1995; **23**, 964–72.

Hayes JA, Black NA, Jenkinson C *et al.* Outcome measures for adult critical care: a systematic review. *Health Technology Assessment* 2000; **4**, 1–111.

Horowitz M, Wilner N, Alvarez W Impact of Events Scale: a measure of subjective distress. *Psychosomatic Medicine* 1979; **41**, 209–18.

Hunt SM, McEwen J, McKenna SP Measuring health status: a new tool for clinicians and epidemiologists. *Journal of the Royal College of General Practitioners* 1985; **35**, 185–8.

Jennett B, Bond M Assessment of outcome after severe brain damage. *Lancet* 1975; **1**, 480–4.

Katz S, Downs TD, Cash HR, Grotz RC Progress in development of the index of ADL. *Gerontologist* 1970; **10**, 20–30.

Knaus WA, Draper EA, Wagner DP *et al.* APACHE II: A severity of disease classification system. *Critical Care Medicine* 1985; **13**, 818–29.

Knaus WA, Draper EA, Wagner DP, Zimmerman JE An evaluation of outcome from intensive care in major medical centers. *Annals of Internal Medicine* 1986; **104**, 410–18.

Knaus WA, Wagner DP, Draper EA *et al.* The APACHE III Prognostic System: risk prediction of hospital mortality for critically ill hospitalized adults. *Chest* 1991; **100**, 1619–36.

Lam S, Ridley S Critically ill medical patients, their demographics and outcome. *Anaesthesia* 1999; **54**, 845–52.

Le Gall JR, Lemeshow S, Saulnier F A new Simplified Acute Physiology Score (SAPS II) based on a European/North American multicenter study. *Journal of the American Medical Association* 1993; **270**, 2957–63.

Lemeshow S, Teres D, Klar J *et al.* Mortality Probability Models (MPM II) based on an international cohort of intensive care unit patients. *Journal of the American Medical Association* 1993; **270**, 2478–86.

McNair DM, Lorr M, Droppleman LF *EdITS Manual for the Profile of Mood States.* Educational and Industrial Testing Service, San Diego: 1992.

Moreno R, Agthe D ICU discharge decision-making: are we able to decrease post-ICU mortality? *Intensive Care Medicine* 1999; **25**, 1035–6.

Pollack MM, Ruttimann UE, Getson PR Pediatric risk of mortality (PRISM) score. *Critical Care Medicine* 1988; **16**, 1110–16.

Ridley SA *Outcomes in Critical Care.* Butterworth-Heinemann, Oxford: 2002.

Ridley SA, Plenderleith L Survival after intensive care. Comparison with a matched normal population as an indicator of effectiveness. *Anaesthesia* 1994; **49**, 933–5.

Rockwood K, Noseworthy TW, Gibney RT *et al.* One-year outcome of elderly and young patients admitted to intensive care units. *Critical Care Medicine* 1993; **21**, 687–91.

Vincent JL, Moreno R, Takala J *et al.* The SOFA (Sepsis-related Organ Failure Assessment) score to describe organ dysfunction/failure. On behalf of the Working Group on Sepsis-related Problems of the European Society of Intensive Care Medicine. *Intensive Care Medicine* 1996; **22**, 707–10.

Ware MK, Snow KK, Kosinski M, Gandek B. *SF-36 Health survey: Manual and interpretation Guide.* The Health Institute, New England Medical Center, Boston, MA: 1993.

Wu AW, Damiano AM, Lynn J *et al.* Predicting future functional status for seriously ill hospitalized adults. The SUPPORT prognostic model. *Annals of Internal Medicine* 1995; **122**, 342–50.

Zigmond AS, Snaith RP The Hospital Anxiety and Depression Scale. *Acta Psychiatrica Scandinavica* 1983; **67**, 361–70.

Clinical supervision: supporting staff and raising standards

Carolyn Temple and Maire Shelly

Introduction

While clinical supervision is applied in various ways, there is a common underlying theme. Supervision is 'a formal process of professional support and learning which enables individual practitioners to develop knowledge and competence, assume responsibility for their own practice and enhance consumer protection and safety of care in complex clinical situations' (Department of Health, 1993). Fundamentally, then, clinical supervision is a process of education that aims to improve the quality of a service. Although further investigation into the effectiveness of clinical supervision is important, available evidence suggests that it does, indeed, improve patient outcome and that lack of supervision is detrimental (McKee and Black, 1992; Fallon *et al.*, 1993; Gennis and Gennis, 1993; Sox *et al.*, 1998).

Although the overall aim of clinical supervision and appraisal is the same, to improve the quality of care provided in a service, the approaches are different. Appraisal is a formal process carried out by peers within a given framework. The main objective of appraisal is to satisfy the management of the organization that practice is safe and that recognized standards are being met. For consultants working in the NHS, appraisal is compulsory from April 2001.

Clinical supervision may be set up and supported within the management framework of an organization. It differs fundamentally from appraisal by creating the opportunity for clinicians and teams to reflect on their practice and for them to set the agenda, a bottom up approach rather than the top down approach to appraisal. The two processes can be seen as complementary and clinicians who participate in meaningful clinical supervision can really make it work for them. They can explore their areas of vulnerability and development needs in clinical supervision and then approach the appraisal process with increased confidence and effectiveness.

Because of its team approach, critical care is an ideal field in which to use clinical supervision as a model to develop and improve clinical practice. Follow-up clinics are a relatively new initiative for most intensive care units (ICU) and are important in this area for two main reasons. First, the quality of care delivered by follow-up clinics requires consideration. They deal with an area in which the psychological and emotional support of patients and their families is as important as the physical support. Staff need education and support so they are able to deal with these areas effectively. Secondly, a follow-up clinic is an invaluable opportunity to assess the quality of care provided on an ICU. It, therefore, acts as a source of feedback to the ICU staff.

In this chapter, we will outline the historical context in which clinical supervision has developed to become established practice in many areas of the health service. We will also set out the principles on which clinical supervision is based and apply these to critical care. We will then suggest a way in which clinical supervision can be introduced into the service and describe the conditions necessary within an organization for effective clinical supervision to flourish.

Historical context

Some health services, for instance mental health and midwifery, have had well-established supervision as an integral part of their delivery for over 30 years. Nursing staff forms the majority of healthcare professionals and over the last 10 years there has been a national drive to establish clinical supervision for nurses (Bishop, 1994).

The recent government initiative of clinical governance and an ever-increasing doubt in the public perception that professional bodies can self-regulate, have made organizations and professional groups consider how best they can create an environment in which clinical excellence will be aspired to by all clinicians and managers. Clinical governance has many facets including quality, standards, life-long learning, professional self-regulation and developing an effective work-force. It can be defined as 'a framework through which NHS organisations are accountable for continuously improving the quality of their services and safeguarding high standards of care' (Department of Health, 1998). Clinical governance places responsibility for the quality of care on organizations and it is the means by which organizations ensure they provide this quality care by making individuals accountable for setting, maintaining and monitoring performance standards.

The changes in the delivery of critical care proposed in Comprehensive Critical Care (Department of Health, 2000) are profound. In order to implement these changes, strategies for education, training, quality assurance and pro-fessional development must be built in; clinical supervision can have a key role in this process.

Principles of clinical supervision

Clinical supervision is one of several strategies that can support performance management within the clinical governance agenda. The more formal management-led strategies for performance management range from disciplinary action, management supervision, preceptorship (the formal induction process within nursing) and management-led appraisal systems. Clinical supervision and mentorship have a clinical rather than managerial basis where the individual or the clinical team lead the process and set the agenda. Performance management itself is outside the remit of this chapter but further details are available (Northcott, 2000).

Clinical supervision is a personal and professional development tool with three functions that are mutually inclusive (Kadushin, 1976; Proctor, 1987). These three functions are reflected across professions (Kadushin, 1976; Johns, 1993; Brocklehurst, 1997; Crespi and Fischetti, 1997; Coles, 1998).

- Educational: this is about developing the skills and understanding the general abilities of the supervisee, developing their awareness of why and how interventions are used and exploring alternative strategies while ensuring that practice is evidence-based.
- Managerial: this is related to the qualitative aspects of the work the supervisee undertakes. The qualitative aspect of supervision is concerned with issues related to equity and fairness to colleagues and to the organization as a whole. Managerial supervision is not about making judgements on people and their work but about highlighting areas for improvement and change of which the supervisee may not be fully aware.
- Supportive: this is a way of responding to supervisees as individuals who are working with people who have complex needs. Supervisees should be encouraged to reflect on ways in which they have been affected by their experiences and they may, as a result, relate differently to others.

Clinical supervision in critical care

Clinical supervision is a model that can be applied to all healthcare professions working within the concept of clinical governance. It includes elements of teaching and mentorship and goes beyond a pastoral role to enable the supervisee to improve their practice. In critical care, supervision is established in particular areas, such as the educational supervision of medical trainees and the mentoring of nursing staff. The concept of clinical supervision builds on this experience and provides supervision for all.

The development of critical care (Department of Health, 2000) will introduce new aspects of practice, such as outreach and patient follow-up, that will necessitate training of staff so that they can deliver care effectively. The document, *Comprehensive Critical Care* (Department of Health, 2000) suggests that training will need to focus on the acutely ill patient and to address the provision of 'pastoral care and psychological support to patients and relatives'. In follow-up clinics and bereavement services, such a focus is vital. Supervision is already an essential part of other services where psychological support is given, for example counselling and psychotherapy. Critical care should not ignore the importance of effective supervision in the delivery of such a service (Harkness and Hensley, 1991; Watkins, 1993, 1994; Goodyear and Bernard, 1998).

The follow-up clinic is also a source of feedback from patients and their families for other staff working in critical care areas. Clinical supervision provides a model whereby this feedback can be used constructively to improve the quality of care delivered in these areas. The links with outreach care, the multiprofessional nature of critical care teams and the liaison with other teams, are all able to enhance the service in different ways.

The culture of quality

For clinical supervision to work, as with appraisal and other performance management strategies, the overall culture of the organization, 'how things are done around here' (Egan, 1994), has to appreciate and invest in quality care. The culture of the Trust or of the ICU will have a powerful impact on how clinical supervision is perceived and valued by staff. A Trust that aspires to being a 'learning organization' is one in which growth, development and learning are all central. Performance management is seen as an essential tool with which to develop the culture and it has been used as a proactive strategy for developing both the staff and the organization collaboratively. The sort of organization that supports such collaborative development will have a culture with values such as those listed in Table 15.1.

The quality agenda requires that most organizations change their culture. This requires strong leadership from Trust Chief Executives and senior managers as

Table 15.1 Some values of an organization supportive of clinical supervision

---

- Learning is a life-long activity for all staff
- All work situations have the potential to create learning opportunities
- Problems are learning opportunities
- Good practice comes from learning and developing competence
- Feedback is on-going and constructive and at all levels
- Change takes time
- Regular review and evaluation are important for both the individual and the organization

---

well as those who lead professional groups. Clinical supervision can be used to support this change in culture.

Clinical supervision in practice

When clinical supervision is introduced into a service area or throughout an organization, it has its best chance of becoming firmly established in the culture of the organization when there is collaboration between staff and managers. Clinical supervision can then become an essential and fundamental component of both delivering and developing high quality clinical services. Services that can be valued by staff and managers alike and where there is tangible evidence of effectiveness.

A commitment to clinical supervision at the most senior level within the organization is essential. Trust Boards must be persuaded that the investment in time and people to provide clinical supervision will be value for money. Some of the benefits that can be observed and monitored in a critical care context are outlined in Table 15.2. Nurturing and encouraging a culture of openness within an organization can improve risk management. Such a culture would regard critical incident reporting as an important opportunity to learn so that similar events can be prevented in the future.

Table 15.2 Observable benefits of clinical supervision in critical care at organizational level

- Improved outcomes of clinical care for patients
- Reduced staff sickness and absence
- Improved staff recruitment and retention
- Reduced numbers of complaints
- Improved risk management

Table 15.3 Different ways to organize the process of clinical supervision

- One-to-one supervision with a supervisor from the same profession
- One-to-one supervision with a supervisor from a different profession
- Group supervision. This is where a group or team have supervision together and may be uniprofessional or multiprofessional. The recommended ratio of supervisor to supervisees is 1:4–5; if the group is larger, this may mean using two supervisors or splitting the group
- Network supervision. This is a type of group supervision where the group members have similar expertise and interests but do not work together on a day-to-day basis

There is a need to respect individuality when rolling out a clinical supervision programme within a Trust or within a department. There are a variety of ways of organizing the process while the basic principles are upheld; these are detailed in Table 15.3 (Kilminister and Jolly, 2000). The ways of organizing the process can be flexibly applied, so that different departments within a Trust have different systems of clinical supervision but all have the same aim.

In the medical profession, most supervision occurs on a one-to-one basis and its primary focus is educational rather than clinical. Critical care is a multidisciplinary and multiprofessional speciality and as such, may lend itself to multiprofessional group supervision. The group could, for instance, reflect on specific interactions with patients or their families or on decision-making processes, such as about withdrawing or withholding care. Multiprofessional group supervision can provide a framework in which differing views can be expressed. By working through real issues, members of the group can reflect on and challenge their own beliefs and decisions. This in turn, can lead to changes in the culture with agreement about the approach to care and with new standards being set for the future that can be audited.

The supervisors are vital to the success of the process. They should be experienced practitioners with clinical credibility who are able to demonstrate the qualities outlined in Table 15.4 (Cote, 1993; Challis *et al.*, 1998; Eaton *et al.*, 1998). Trusts have a responsibility to provide training to appropriately experienced practitioners who are willing to undertake the role of supervisor. Supervisors should receive clinical supervision themselves either on a one-to-one basis or in a small group. The roles of a supervisor are detailed in Table 15.5.

The relationship of the supervisor with the supervisee is crucial to the success of clinical supervision (Harkness, 1995; Kilminister and Jolly, 2000). Self-supervision does not improve care as supervision by another does (Skeff *et al.*, 1997). The relationship between the supervisor and the supervisee should be dynamic and able to change as the needs of the supervisee change (Nolan *et al.*, 1993; Parak *et al.*, 1997). However, evidence suggests that continuity of the

Table 15.4 The qualities of a clinical supervisor

- Good interpersonal and communication skills so that they can give effective feedback on performance and are empathic and supportive in a non-judgemental way
- That they personally apply reflective practice skills
- A professional maturity, i.e. a willingness, openness and confidence to challenge practice issues
- That they understand the issues of personal accountability and responsibility and are able to delegate responsibility to others
- An up-to-date knowledge base in the relevant field and clinical credibility
- If necessary, that they have teaching, facilitation, negotiation and counselling skills and a knowledge of learning opportunities and requirements

---

Table 15.5 The roles of a supervisor

- Ensure protected time for each supervisee to lay out issues in his or her own way
- Help supervisees explore and clarify their thinking, feeling and underlying beliefs about their practice
- Enable supervisees to identify and discuss critical incidents and/or stressful aspects of their professional work
- Share experience, information and skills appropriately
- Challenge practice that they perceive as unethical, unwise or incompetent
- Challenge personal and professional blindspots which they may perceive in individuals or in the group
- Be aware of the organizational contracts that they and the supervisees may have with the employer and clients in terms of supervision
- Facilitate professional development

---

relationship over time is important to the success of supervision (Bishop, 1998). Training of supervisors is valuable (Williams and Webb, 1994; Lenton *et al.*, 1994; Peel *et al.*, 1996; Twinn and Davies, 1996; Bishop, 1998); some courses are based on an assessment of educational supervisors' needs (Challis *et al.*, 1998) however, most are not empirically based.

One way of engaging supervisees in the process of clinical supervision is to arrange a session where they can be made aware of the process and agree on how to implement it within their part of the organization (Frame, 2000). This enables the roles of the supervisee (Table 15.6) to be made explicit. Some authors advocate training supervisees as well as supervisors, so that they get the most out of their supervision (Porter, 1997).

The agreement on how to implement clinical supervision may contain practical points and supporting documentation, for example it may contain a contract signed by both the supervisor and supervisee with the agreed frequency, length and venue of the supervision sessions and the planned series of sessions for the year ahead. A confidentiality clause should be included making explicit the limits

Table 15.6 The roles of the supervisee

- To identify practice issues with which they need help and to ask for time to consider alternative approaches
- To become increasingly able to share these issues freely
- To contribute to reflective discussion on clinical practice
- To become more aware of themselves and their relationships with clients, patients, colleagues and the supervisor or supervision group
- To respond to feedback from their supervisor in a structured and professional manner
- To consider their training and development needs

---

of confidentiality, so all parties are aware of when confidentiality can be broken and for what reasons. Agreement should also be reached between the supervisor and supervisee about any documentation of issues discussed within the supervision session and the outcomes of the discussion. This information, once anonymized, may be used to support the monitoring and audit process. The Trust's clinical governance committee will be key in this monitoring and auditing process. They will be able to close the audit loop by identifying evidence of changes in practice as a result of the investment by the Trust in the time and training to support this activity.

Conclusion

The proposed changes in the delivery of critical care are a real opportunity to introduce clinical supervision into critical care. In this way service development can mirror professional development and quality can be assured in both.

References

Bishop V Clinical supervision for an accountable profession. *Nursing Times* 1994; **90**, 35–7.

Bishop V (ed.) *Clinical Supervision in Practice, Some Questions Answers and Guidelines.* Macmillan Press, Basingstoke: 1998.

Brocklehurst N Clinical supervision in nursing homes. *Nursing Times* 1997; **93**, 48–9.

Challis M, Williams J, Batstone G Supporting pre-registration house officers: the needs of educational supervisors of the first phase of the post-graduate medical education. *Medical Education* 1998; **32**, 177–80.

Coles C The educational supervisor's role in medicine. In: (Peyton JWR, ed.) *Teaching & Learning in Medical Practice.* Manticore Europe Ltd, Heronsgate, Rickmansworth, Herts: 1998, pp 117–27.

Cote L Supervision of family medicine residents. *Canadian Family Physician* 1993; **39**, 366–72.

Crespi TD, Fischetti BA Clinical supervision for school psychologists. *School of Psychological Interventions* 1997; **18**, 41–8.

Department of Health *A Vision for the Future: the Nursing, Midwifery and Health Visiting Contribution to Health Care.* HMSO, London: 1993.

Department of Health *A First Class Service – Quality in the New NHS.* HMSO, London: 1998.

Department of Health *Comprehensive Critical Care. a Review of Adult Critical Care Services.* HMSO, London: 2000.

Eaton J, Coles C, Buckle L *Educational Supervision.* Departments of Post Graduate Medical and Dental Education South and West, Bristol: 1998.

Egan G Cultivate your culture. *Management Today* 1994; April, 38–42.

Fallon WF Jr, Wears RL, Tepas JJ 3rd Resident supervision in the operating room: does this impact on outcome? *Journal of Trauma* 1993; **35**, 556–61.

Frame G *A Charter for Clinical Supervision*. Chester and Halton Community NHS Trust, 2000.

Gennis VM, Gennis MA Supervision in the outpatient clinic: effects on teaching and patient care. *Journal of General Internal Medicine* 1993; **8**: 378–80.

Goodyear RK, Bernard JM Clinical supervision: lessons from the literature. *Counselling and Education Supplement* 1998; **38**, 6–22.

Harkness D, Hensley H Changing the focus of social work supervision: effects on client satisfaction and generalized contentment. *Social Work* 1991; **36**, 506–12.

Harkness D The art of helping in supervised practice. Skills, relationships, outcomes. *Clinical Supervisor* 1995; **13**, 63–76.

Johns C Professional supervision. *Journal of Nursing Management* 1993; **1**, 9–18.

Kadushin A *Supervision in Social Work*. Columbia University Press, New York and London: 1976.

Kilminster SM, Jolly BC Effective supervision in clinical practice settings: a literature review. *Medical Education* 2000; **34**, 827–40.

Lenton SW, Dison PJ, Haines LC A BPA survey of recently appointed consultants. *Archives of Disease in Childhood* 1994; **71**, 381–5.

McKee M, Black N Does the current use of junior doctors in the United Kingdom affect the quality of medical care. *Social Science Medicine* 1992; **34**, 549–58.

Nolan J, Hawkes B, Francis P Case studies: windows into clinical supervision. *Educational Leadership* 1993; **51**, 52–6.

Northcott N Clinical supervision – Professional development or management control? In: (Spouse J, Redfern L, eds). *Successful Supervision in Health Care Practice – Promoting Professional Development*. Blackwell Science, Oxford: 2000, pp 10–29.

Parak M, Pearlman-Avnion S, Glanz J Using developmental supervision to improve science and technology instruction in Israel. *Journal of Curriculum and Supervision* 1997; **12**, 367–82.

Peel ALG, Ramsden PD, Proud G MRCS training: plans for a regional day release training scheme. *Annals of the Royal College of Surgeons of England* 1996; **78** (Suppl. 5), 221–2.

Porter N Clinical supervision: the art of being supervised. *Nursing Standard* 1997; **11**, 44–5.

Proctor B Supervision. A co-operative exercise in accountability. In: (Marken M, Payne M, eds). *Enabling and Ensuring Supervision in Practice*. National Youth Bureau and Council for Education and Training in Youth and Community Work, Leicester: 1987.

Skeff KM, Bowen JL, lrby DM Protecting time for teaching in the ambulatory care setting. *Academic Medicine* 1997; **72**, 694–7.

Sox CM, Burstin HR, Orav EJ *et al*. The effect of supervision of residents on quality of care in five university-affiliated emergency departments. *Academic Medicine* 1998; **73**, 776–82.

Twinn S, Davies S The supervision of Project 2000 students in the clinical setting: issues and implications for practitioners. *Journal of Clinical Nursing* 1996; **5**, 177–83.

Watkins CE Jr Development of the psychotherapy supervisors: concepts, assumptions, and hypotheses of the supervisors complexity model. *American Journal of Psychotherapy* 1993; **47**, 58–74.

Watkins CE Jr The supervision of psychotherapy supervisors trainees. *American Journal of Psychotherapy* 1994; **48**, 417–31.

Williams PL, Webb C Clinical supervision skills: a Delphi and critical incident technique study. *Medical Teaching* 1994; **16**, 139–57.

Index